HEARING THERAPY
for CHILDREN

SECOND, REVISED EDITION

ALICE STRENG, M.A.

WARING J. FITCH, M.A.

LeROY D. HEDGECOCK, Ph.D.

JAMES W. PHILLIPS, M.D.

JAMES A. CARRELL, Ph.D.

617.8
St8h

Grune & Stratton   1958
New York   London

THE AUTHORS

ALICE STRENG is Chairman, Department of Exceptional Education, University of Wisconsin, Milwaukee.

WARING J. FITCH is Hearing Consultant, Washington State Department of Health; Lecturer,. University of Washington.

LeROY D. HEDGECOCK is Consulting Audiologist, Mayo Clinic.

JAMES W. PHILLIPS is Otolaryngologist in Private Practice; Consultant, Washington State Department of Health; Lecturer, University of Washington.

JAMES A. CARRELL is Director, Speech and Hearing Clinic, University of Washington.

Library of Congress Catalog Card No. 58–11706

First Edition copyright © 1955
and
Second Edition copyright © 1958
GRUNE & STRATTON, INC.
381 Fourth Avenue
New York City 16

Printed and Bound in U. S. A.

(B)

Contents

1117497

PREFACE TO THE SECOND EDITION

IN PREPARING a revision of *Hearing Therapy for Children* the authors have undertaken to correct occasional errors, provide clearer discussion of certain points and make numerous other changes while retaining the basic format and content of the first edition. We should like to express our gratitude for the reception the book has received and we continue to hope that our efforts will be of some small use to all who are concerned in one way or another with the problems of the children about whom we have written.

THE AUTHORS

PREFACE TO THE FIRST EDITION

WHAT goes on in the mind of a young child who is shut out of the hearing world? It is not altogether accurate to say the same thoughts and concepts as are found in any child's mind. So many of our thought processes depend on what we hear, and for such a child the auditory clues are lacking. If we might follow the workings of his mind, we would find that it is his eyes that tell him what is going on, eyes that sometimes see a hostile, impatient world. He sees something interesting but he cannot say, "What is it?" or "May I have it?" He does not have the speech and language. Instead he must pick it up, feel it, put it in his mouth. This finding-out process may bring him into conflict with his world, especially if the object is a sharp knife, a piece of fine china or a flickering candle.

If he is partially deaf, contact with his world will include some auditory clues—a kind of partial, inaccurate blur of sound. He may have speech, but it is likely to be defective and difficult to understand. His world too may be one of many frustrations.

What people make up the world of a hearing handicapped child? Parents, brothers and sisters know him best, but they may need help in understanding his problem. Even though resourceful and well-meaning, parents often have feelings about the child which stand in the way of their helping. The physician who examines the child, the public health nurse who visits his home, the speech and hearing therapist, special class or regular class teacher, social worker and school administrator all share various degrees of responsibility in developing educational facilities and promoting understanding.

The chapters which follow are designed to include for the first time in one book the special skills and knowledge needed by members of those professional groups who work with hearing handicapped children.

THE AUTHORS

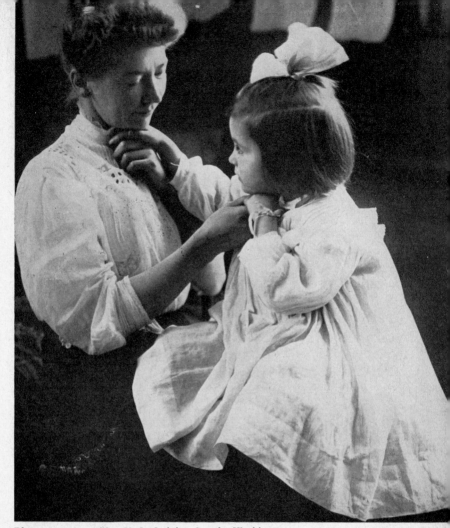

Photo courtesy of Mrs. H. L. Quigley, Seattle, Washington

Introduction

Deafness Then and Now

A VISITOR to an Eastern city a century ago was shown a building of darkly imposing architecture. ASYLUM FOR THE DEAF AND DUMB was chiseled in stone over its entrance. "What a pity! those poor blighted young lives," the visitor said. They were indeed to be pitied, because these children were among the legion of poorly understood, rejected youngsters for whom society had no place and no hope. Frequently the blind, crippled, mentally defective, emotionally disturbed and deaf children were housed together, without regard for their various needs. Asylum, a term meaning place of refuge, was most appropriate since all these children needed protection from the cruel jokes, ridicule, rejection or unenlightened sympathy in the world outside.

Today a visitor to the same city might be shown a shining modern school to which the deaf and hard of hearing children of the community come each morning, along with their playmates—the "normal children." Within would be found not only the classrooms one would expect in any modern school, but also special rooms planned and equipped for the needs of the acoustically handicapped youngsters. Their instruction would follow the lines laid out by many years of experience and extensive research on the education of the deaf and hard of hearing child. If our visitor were to observe the children at recess—in the sandbox, on the swings, absorbed in a clamorous game of tag or kick-ball—he might well inquire, "Which of these children are deaf?"

If he were to follow these children as they grow and learn through the years he would discover that they are no longer the forgotten children, living out their days without hope. Through modern medical and educational techniques these youngsters acquire the same basic learning skills and information they would have acquired if they had not been deaf or hard of hearing. They read, write, understand—perhaps by lip reading—and they even speak; and when they are finally graduated, some perhaps with a college degree, they are prepared to take their places in society as productive workers and good citizens. What is less tangible, but of vast importance, is that they are less likely to be thought of as "handicapped," but rather as persons with their own pattern of assets and liabilities who nevertheless find themselves leading happy, useful lives.

All this has not come about quickly or easily, nor have the opportunities for training and education been made available to all who need them. The transition in status of the acoustically handicapped during the past century has been slow and difficult. The fortunate deaf adults of today live rich and useful lives with their hearing contemporaries. But there are still uncounted numbers whose opportunities have been limited and who constitute a tremendous waste of human resources. Quite clearly, this situation must be corrected by marshalling further the energies of all who are concerned—our doctors, teachers, parents, public health nurses, community leaders and others.

Some knowledge of the history of the management of problems of the acoustically handicapped will be helpful in interpreting modern practices and procedures. In very early times the deaf were regarded with much superstition, and were sometimes even put to death, classed with the insane or treated otherwise in conformity with primitive mores. One of the first recorded accounts of the education of the deaf tells of the success of St. John of Beverly in teaching a deaf mute to speak in about the year 700 A. D. In the 16th century Jerome Cardan, of Pavia, put forth the premise that the deaf could be taught by writing. Pedro Ponce, a Benedictine monk, is said to have used this method with success.

Another Spanish monk, Juan Paulo Bonet, in 1620 published a book on his experience in teaching the deaf. In England meanwhile, about 1643, Dr. John Bulwer also wrote a book on teaching the "deaf and dumb." In 1680 a Scotsman, George Dalgarno, published a volume titled *Deaf and Dumb Man's Tutor*. A century later Thomas Braidwood opened a school for the deaf in Edinburgh and Abbé de l'Eppe established a similar institution in Paris. In 1793 Braidwood founded the Asylum for the Deaf and Dumb in London.

In the United States the first attempt to teach a deaf mute of which we have record was at Rowley, Massachusetts, in 1679. It was not until the early 19th century, however, that much was done in this country to educate deaf children. In 1803 a group of ministers in Massachusetts made a census of the deaf and found 75 in their state. They estimated there were 500 deaf persons in the United States and set about to establish a special school for their training. At about the same time a New York City minister, John Stanford, found several deaf children in almshouses and undertook to teach them. In 1812 John Braidwood, a grandson of Thomas Braidwood, taught a family of deaf children in Virginia. He subsequently established a school, but this was discontinued after his death for want of a teacher.

Shortly thereafter occurred one of the most significant series of events in the history of the education of the deaf in the United States. In Hartford, Connecticut, young Alice Cogswell, daughter of a physician, attracted the sympathetic interest of a group of local citizens because she did not hear. Aroused to the problem, these community leaders sought other deaf children and found 84 within the state. They estimated there were 400 deaf individuals in New England. Moved to action, they founded a society in 1815 to instruct the deaf and took the very practical step of raising the sum of $2,278 which was used to send a young minister, the Reverend Thomas H. Gallaudet, abroad to learn methods of teaching the deaf. He studied "sign language" in Paris for a year and upon his return to Hartford the American Asylum for the Deaf was opened there in 1817. Children from all parts of the country attended the new school. The following year a similar school was started in New York, another was founded in Philadelphia in 1820 and soon thereafter others opened their doors elsewhere. The movement to provide education for the deaf was truly on its way, although the curricula were limited as compared to those of today and all instruction was carried out in the manual language.

Three decades later the distinguished Alexander Melville Bell and his even more distinguished son, Alexander Graham Bell, became a powerful influence in the history of the education of the deaf in the United States. The elder Bell, who was a well-known English scientist and student of voice physiology, was in this country on a lecture tour, leaving his son in charge of professional duties at home in England. The father, Alexander Melville Bell, had devised an ingenious method of recording the position of the speech articulators in talking which he called "Visible Speech." This system of symbols, he told his interested American audience, had been successfully adapted by his son to the instruction of deaf children in a school at Kensington.

As a result of the interest aroused by the elder Bell's lecture the Boston School Board in 1869 opened a special day school for the deaf—the first of its kind—and placed Miss Sarah Fuller in charge. Having heard Alexander Melville Bell's lecture, she persuaded her employers to invite the young Alexander Graham Bell to come to Boston to train her teachers in the methods which he was using with such success with the deaf children of England. He arrived at Miss Fuller's school in April of 1871. The system of Visible Speech which he brought with him is even today the basis for the method used in teaching the deaf to talk.

Bell completed his course for the Boston teachers in three months, visited other schools for a time, and in October, 1872, opened a private class in Boston for teachers of the deaf to which various schools and institutions sent their instructors for training in Visible Speech. The following year Alexander Graham Bell, then twenty-five years of age, was appointed to the faculty of Boston University where he started a teacher-training class. At night and in odd hours the young teacher-scientist worked tirelessly on a kind of "electric speaking telegraph" which he hoped would eventually show his young pupils how to express their voice tone vibrations properly.

In 1877 Bell married Mabel G. Hubbard, daughter of his close friend who was a founder of the National Geographic Society. As a child of three Mabel Hubbard had become deaf through scarlet fever. Because of his concern for the deaf, aroused by his own deaf youngster, Hubbard led a movement which resulted in founding the Clarke Institute for Deaf Mutes at Northampton, Massachusetts in 1867. This school, later renamed and still existing as the Clarke School for the Deaf, was the first permanent American school to use the oral method of instruction, as contrasted to the "sign language." Another oral school, The Institution for Improved Instruction of the Deaf, now the Lexington School for the Deaf, was opened in New York City on about this same date.

Since these beginnings, enormous progress has been made possible by the growth of facilities for early discovery and medical treatment of the child with a hearing disorder. Through research and clinical experience, coupled with the development of new drugs, the otologist has learned to treat successfully many of the ear diseases which formerly could not be reached. The result has been fewer permanent hearing losses; in other cases where hearing cannot be restored to normal the defect frequently can be made less severe.

Equally gratifying has been the growth of educational facilities for these children. Today most states maintain a residence school for the deaf, and public schools in major cities commonly provide day classes for children with all degrees of impaired hearing. Many teacher education institutions are cooperating by providing the highly specialized training for teachers for these children. Although public understanding and acceptance of the deaf are at high level, there is still much ground to be gained. The following incident was observed by Miss Mildred Groht, Principal of the Lexington School in New York City, as she approached the school one day. In front of her was a small boy, possibly four years old, and with him was a woman who apparently was his nurse. The nurse said impressively, "This is where the little deaf and dumb children go to school." Then after a slight pause to let the enormity of this sink in, she continued, "Maybe someday we can see one of them."

The purpose of this book is to provide a report of modern medical and educational procedures which can be applied to help the child with an auditory disorder overcome or minimize his handicap.

BIBLIOGRAPHY

BEST, HARRY: Deafness and the Deaf in the United States. New York, Macmillan, 1941.

DeLAND, FRED: The Story of Lip Reading. Washington, D. C., The Volta Bureau, 1931.

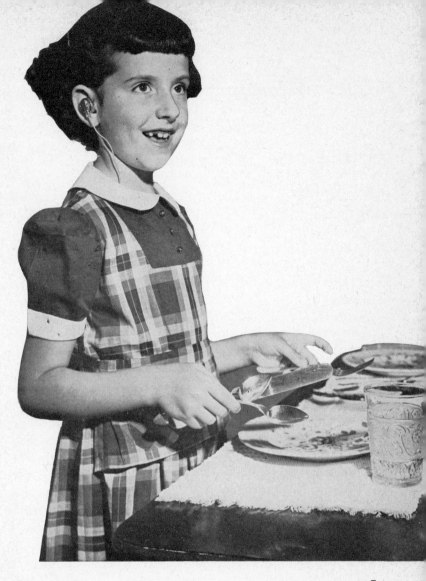

Problems of Deafness in Children

IT IS an oversimplification to say that the child with a hearing disability is like any other child with the exception of his impaired auditory sense. Deafness, in whatever degree, necessarily brings a modification in the total reaction of the individual. In the past, speculations have arisen to the effect that the deaf possess keener visual acuity and sharper powers of observation than do persons with normal hearing. While this has not been experimentally demonstrated, it has a sound underlying premise. It acknowledges that the stability of the individual is threatened by the sensory defect, and the individual thus threatened is challenged to mobilize his remaining resources more effectively. He develops compensatory skills in order to meet the demands of his environment. Furthermore, this view assumes that the sense of hearing is inseparably integrated with the total individual. The absence of hearing must involve a reorganization of his entire dynamic system, causing him to behave in a qualitatively different manner in order that he may adjust and survive.[1]

Psychologically there is a difference between a child with five senses and one with four. All our knowledge and experience are gained through the channels of the five senses, and if one of these avenues is closed there is a difference in the sum total of the individual's mental content. This does not necessarily mean that a deaf child is inferior to a hearing child, but it implies that the mental development would have been fuller and more evenly balanced had he possessed an adequate sense of hearing.[2]

In the normal child, hearing and vision work together in a complementary relationship as distance senses. Vision is directed to the foreground and hearing encompasses the background as well as the entire environment. Vision is directional, relating the child to those objects and activities immediately before him, and to a limited degree on either side. Hearing is nondirectional, extending to the total environment, functioning night and day, around corners and into the dark. For the child who does not hear normally, vision must serve perceptively in both foreground and background. Many hearing handicapped children develop a kinesthetic sense, an awareness more highly developed than in hearing children. Footsteps are felt and vision directed. Thus, the deaf child utilizes kinesthetic and visual senses in place of hearing and vision. There are obvious limitations to this combination, making it difficult for the child to keep in touch with his environment, to explore it and to know it fully. When a visual experience is not supplemented by the accompanying auditory experience, the visual experience is different.[3]

In the normal child, an intersensory perception provides him with an understanding and interpretation of his sensory experiences. The visual, tactile, olfactory, auditory and other senses work in a complementary relationship to give him a full perception. The child with defective hearing is denied, in some degree, the auditory ingredient, thus modifying and limiting his total sensory experience.

DEFINITIONS

The child who is born with little or no hearing, or who has suffered the loss early in infancy before speech and language patterns are acquired is said to be deaf. One who is born with normal hearing and reaches the age where he can produce and comprehend speech but subsequently loses his hearing is described as deafened. The hard of hearing are those with reduced hearing acuity either since birth or acquired at any time during life.

EFFECTS OF DEAFNESS

The effects of deafness, a cutting off of auditory stimulation, are more or less uniform regardless of the cause. There are certain important variants: the age of onset, degree of deafness and whether the onset was gradual or sudden. The child who loses his hearing at the age of four or five, after he has acquired speech and language, obviously will not be as handicapped as the child of the same age who has never heard. Since hearing loss may range quantitatively from slight to severe, it is axiomatic that the greater the loss the greater the handicap. Losses of sudden onset from accident or disease may have a profound effect on the personality of the child.

The deaf baby is no different from any other baby during his first few months of life. He is not dumb or mute as was mistakenly believed in the past. He has a voice, he babbles, coos, cries, laughs and makes all the sounds that hearing babies make, but because he cannot hear his own voice these sounds will not develop naturally into speech.[4]

For many babies the first suspicion of deafness comes when the infant is 12 to 18 months of age, or earlier. He fails to look toward his mother as she speaks to him, he does not react to loud sounds, and his own vocalization remains at the babbling stage rather than developing into purposeful sounds to which his parents respond. At this time the parents may take him to the baby specialist or family physician only to be told that there is nothing wrong, that all babies do not sit up, walk or talk at the same age, and when the baby is ready to talk he will talk. Perhaps a few more months pass. The baby's physical growth pattern is normal, and since communication in infancy depends largely on physical contact, facial expression and the baby's sense of well-being, the parents do not always suspect a hearing loss.

It has been cited that the period between suspecting deafness and having the deafness confirmed is probably one of the most frightening emotional periods for both parents. They have little if any knowledge of deafness and what can be done for the deaf child. Consequently, they have visions of their child going through life unable to speak, different from others, a social outcast and a burden. Before the diagnosis is established by the family physician or otologist and accepted by the parents, they may travel from one physician's office to another seeking help, sometimes from one city to another. They may get a number of varied opinions which add to the problem. Or, in spite of getting the same statement from each doctor, they may refuse to face the facts and continue to search for some person who will tell them what they want to hear, that their child is perfectly normal. What is happening to the child as he is being taken from specialist to specialist in the midst of this turmoil of unhappy feelings? Are the parents really thinking of the child or are they seeking relief for themselves?[5]

When they finally learn for certain that their child cannot hear, parents may be precipitated into an emotional upheaval. The impact frequently brings a confusion in which they see only the deafness and not the child. As the shock subsides, both father and mother may need help in adjusting their feelings toward the child. Either consciously or unconsciously there may be feelings of self-reproach, bewilderment or despair for having produced this defective child. Feelings of rejection or hostility are not uncommon, since the deafness with its supposed limitations voids any ambitions they may have had for the child. Serious responsibility rests with the physician in interpreting the problems of deafness realistically, and at the same time hopefully.[6] Referral by him to an appropriate agency in or near the community may be the first step in building hope and assurance for the parents.

There are numerous agencies, both official and voluntary, which are given over to the welfare and education of the deaf and hard of hearing. Official agencies may include state and local departments of health, state and local departments of education, rehabilitation programs and university and college speech and hearing clinics. Voluntary agencies, those supported with funds other than tax money, include children's hospitals, the American Hearing Society, with local chapters in major cities, the John Tracy Clinic, the Volta Bureau, local preschool classes for the deaf, and many others (see Appendix, page 345).

It is significant that most agencies have classes or literature directed toward the parents, since their first real need is an understanding of themselves in relation to the child. Speech and language are not needed to convey feelings of hostility, not even to a little baby. Association with the resourceful parents of other young deaf children, a visit to a class for the deaf, or reading some of the current literature may be reassuring and may begin to bring the child with his deafness into proper focus.

DEAFNESS: A COMMUNICATIVE HANDICAP

The basic problem which concerns any young child with a hearing loss is communication. He does not hear normally, thus he is incapable of fully understanding the spoken language of others. Since he does not understand language, he cannot develop normal communication unless he is trained to do so. He may convey his wants through gesture, facial expression or cries, but speech and language, the substance of communication, fail to develop at the appropriate age levels, as in a child with normal hearing. Also, we have difficulty establishing contact with him since what we say depends largely on auditory symbols which are meaningless to him.

One investigator considers deafness as both a communicative handicap and a sensory defect. The young deaf child can learn to talk intelligibly, but when he speaks he is carrying out an act in which he cannot experience the full sensory effect. He can be taught to read lips, and in doing so he learns to understand a visual pattern of speech without the full auditory sensation. The deaf child, because he must be taught language, begins to learn it at a later date than a normal child, perhaps at a time when the greatest readiness for language acquisition is past, and without the emotionally tinged auditory experience which comes to the normal child without any effort on his part. Retardation in language understanding is the major part of the communicative handicap, and it may bring the deaf child psychologically into regions of insecurity and conflict. Deafness also seems to bring a certain amount of physical insecurity, but deaf children seem less prone to certain fears than normal children. Possibly this is because tales of imaginary dangers, witches and ghosts are abstractions less likely to be understood by deaf children.[7]

THE FAMILY'S PROBLEM

If the hearing handicapped child is a problem to his family, they most certainly will be a problem for him. Not only his parents and siblings, but the entire neighborhood has some influence on the child. Parents, however, are the greatest influence in the child's life since he lives until early adulthood in the atmosphere created by them. If, because of his deafness, he is overprotected, is exempted from family responsibilities and disciplines or takes a disproportionate amount of his mother's time, his brothers and sisters may understandably develop a feeling of hostility for him. If parents feel they must make constant apology for the child, cover up his hearing defect, or keep him from the public eye he will be well aware of the difference in their treatment of him as compared with their management of his brothers and sisters. When parents can accept unreservedly the child with his deafness, this will be sensed by the child and reflected in the others who make up the family and neighborhood. A large part of any child's sense of security comes from knowing that he is loved and that he really counts for something in the family.

Gesell observed that overt responses in deaf children do not always give reliable clues to inner problems. Frequently they represent some form of defense mechanism the child adapts, often unconsciously, to circumvent a difficult situation, to compensate for inadequacies or to resolve unrecognized mental conflicts.[8]

SOCIAL DEVELOPMENT OF YOUNG DEAF CHILDREN

Research to investigate the social development of preschool deaf children found that when the child enters nursery school at the age of three, he is likely to have already been spoiled by an overindulgent family or neglected by bewildered or rejecting parents. In free play with normally hearing children, these youngsters used few gestures representing the names of objects, and only a limited amount of pantomime. Most of their conversation was carried on by pointing and by the use of the head gestures for *yes* and *no* combined with facial expressions. This investigation found that both deaf and hearing children at the preschool level spent a surprising amount of time boasting and calling attention to themselves, to things they had, or were making or could do. The deaf child could do this adequately by pointing, but limitations were evident since his pointing depended very much on the context of the immediate situation for its meaning. It was difficult for him to refer to something in the other room or at home, or something he expected to do the next day. Real frustrations were evident in the deaf child's imaginary play. As soon as he started something he wanted others to appreciate, it was not always easy without words to make another person see what it was all about. The principal difference between the deaf and hearing was that, among the deaf, play groups were more diffuse and less stable, breaking up constantly, possibly because it is more difficult for a child to lead an activity without clarifying words. This study concludes that the earlier we reach the deaf child, educationally, the nearer we will come to bridging the gap that exists between the deaf and normal child in education and social development.[9]

INTELLIGENCE

When native ability is measured with nonverbal or performance tests of intelligence, deaf and hard of hearing children are not found to be inferior in intelligence to normally hearing children. In an unselected group of acoustically handicapped children, scores on intelligence tests will have approximately the same distribution as a similar group of hearing children. One investigator cites that while the deaf are not intellectually inferior, it is more difficult for them to use their reservoir of potential intelligence in as subtle and abstract a manner as the child who hears.[3]

Pintner reports that the age of onset of deafness has no influence on intelligence. His investigations found that nonlanguage, performance or the Goodenough Draw a Man tests were most accurate in measuring native ability in deaf and hard of hearing children. More than 50 per cent of the hearing defective children tested were found to have IQ's of 90 or above. The Revised Stanford Binet was of little value since it requires the child to have normal hearing. Pintner concludes that there is a large reservoir of fine native ability among the deaf.[10]

Myklebust and Burchard,[11] using the Grace Arthur Performance Scale in a comparison of the intelligence of children with congenital and acquired deafness, found both group to have average intelligence with the difference between the groups small and unreliable. They stress that it is important to recognize that the problem in educating and training a deaf child is not one of dealing with mental retardation.

SOCIAL MATURITY

In social maturity—the extent to which the child learns to care for himself and for others—it is more difficult for hearing handicapped children to make the same gains as children with full hearing acuity. There is some basis for thinking that those children who live at home and attend a special school or class in their home community achieve a higher degree of social maturity than those children who attend a state or private residential school. Streng and Kirk, using the Vineland Social Maturity Scale, found no appreciable difference in the social competence of matched pairs of deaf and hearing children attending a special school for the deaf in their home community.[12] Myklebust and Burchard,[11] also using the Vineland Social Maturity Scale, found deaf children living in a residential school less mature than children living at home and attending a day school. They suggest that deep problems are involved in taking a deaf child of four to six years away from his home. Singled out among his brothers and sisters to be sent away, without an explanation which he can understand, might easily be felt as rejection. The result may be a weakening of early identifications and relationships, and have a marked effect on the personality of the child. There is an unavoidable amount of impersonal relationship in a residential school which makes the social climate very different from the average home. These investigators conclude that the difference in social maturity between deaf children in a day school and those attending a residential school cannot be accounted for on the basis of hearing loss or intelligence. The discrepancy suggests that day schools either train deaf children more successfully to be socially mature or select children who are more socially mature. In a comparison of children with congenital and acquired deafness this investigation found no reliable difference between these two groups, but report the retardation for both groups to be significantly below normal.

PERSONALITY

The area of personality has been the least explored of any phase of the development of the child with hearing disability. Possibly this is because most personality inventories involve extensive use of language, and the language handicap of the child would prevent him from fully comprehending the requirements of the test.

The Brown Personality Inventory for Children, a series of 80 questions answered by *yes* or *no* was given to equated pairs of deaf and hearing children. The deaf received much higher neurotic scores than the hearing group, indicating very poor social adjustment. However, an item analysis of the test revealed that there were certain questions in which the sensory defect itself might have conditioned the response rather than the psychologic make-up of the child. The scores and test items were studied jointly by a group of psychologists and adult deaf. As a result, five of the test items which scored heavily against the deaf were deleted. The items included such questions as "Do you feel that people do not understand you?" or "Have you ever been unable to see or hear for a while?" With the omission of these items, the deaf group scored slightly higher but still were in the poor social adjustment category.[13]

Studies have shown that there is little experimental evidence to support the popular feeling that children with hearing disorders are suspicious or have paranoid tendencies. This feeling has probably grown out of experience with adults sustaining hearing loss in middle life. At present, clinical evidence suggests that all types of adjustment are found in a group of auditory defective children. There is fairly conclusive evidence that as a group they are slightly less emotionally stable and less mature than a comparable group of hearing children.[14]

CHILDREN WITH MULTIPLE HANDICAPS

Loss of hearing in children is not infrequently coupled with other handicapping conditions. As a result, the establishment of an early and complete medical diagnosis is hampered because the hearing loss may not be as obvious as the handicap with which it is associated. Many children with cerebral palsy also suffer auditory disability. The lesion which damaged motor areas of the brain may extend to areas of auditory perception, resulting in a total or partial hearing loss. Thus, the child's speech may be involved because he does not have normal hearing in addition to a lack of motor control in the musculature of the speech mechanism.

The child with cleft lip and palate may suffer loss of hearing. During his early months of life, before corrective surgery of the palate is initiated, and during the two or three years required to complete the process, parts of his hearing mechanism are open to easy assault from disease. The congenital lack of palatal structures makes feeding and swallowing difficult for him. Particles of food or liquid may become lodged in his nose. Fluids, like milk or water, have been known to travel to the middle ear by way of the eustachian tubes. The resulting middle ear infection, if allowed to develop, may erode and impair the function of middle ear structures, and may be further disabling by causing perforation, scarring or thickening of the drum membrane.

Hearing loss in mentally retarded children may not be easy to detect, and diagnostic audiometry difficult to achieve. Where this combination of handicaps is suspected, the child should have the benefit of complete psychometric, psychologic, medical and otologic evaluation before the diagnosis of mental retardation is made. In the past, as a result of insufficient study or misdiagnosis, deaf children of normal mentality have been found in institutions for the feebleminded. Conversely, parents of mentally retarded deaf children have brought pressure to keep their children in schools for the deaf, although the deafness was only slight and not the major problem.

Visual Acuity

The incidence of poor peripheral vision in hearing handicapped children exceeds the incidence in normally hearing children, according to a recent investigation. The report suggests that the severe sensory impairment of deafness modifies the total reaction of the child to his environment and is reflected in the child's other perceptual systems, including vision.[1]

Aphasia

Aphasia may result from damage to the part of the cortex described as Broca's area. Although hearing may be normal, the aphasic child is characterized by a lack of ability to express himself by speech, writing or signs; or he may be unable to comprehend spoken or written language. Aphasia is sometimes associated with deafness, especially where the deafness is due to a brain lesion, and a differential diagnosis in such cases is difficult to establish. It is not uncommon for children with cerebral palsy to have some degree of aphasia as well as auditory involvement. Aphasic children are sometimes found in a class for deaf children, since methods of training aphasics in motor speech patterns and language comprehension are essentially the same as those used with the deaf.

Toward Meeting the Problems of Deafness in Children

Perhaps the first step toward meeting the problems of deafness takes place long before the child is born. For various reasons some babies are unwanted, and there is conscious or unconscious rejection by one or both parents even before the baby is born. When the baby is a few months old and parents discover that he does not hear normally, their feelings may be intensified and become more acute. There are some parents whose sense of values makes it difficult for them to accept a girl when their supreme wish was for a boy, or vice versa. Other parents are openly disappointed because the baby has plain features and straight hair instead of the doll-like face and blonde curls they had imagined. Even if rejection is present to an acute degree, it must be said in fairness to the parents of deaf and hard of hearing children that society itself is often responsible for aggravating the problem. Most parents do accept the child, and where they do have difficulty in doing so, they frequently put forth a great deal of effort to accept the child realistically. Their efforts may be frustrated by some friend or well-meaning relative who dwells on the notion that the child is not normal and perhaps "ought to be put away." Playmates are also inadvertently cruel. Parents frequently report that in spite of their efforts to make the child feel like one of the family and neighborhood group, playmates circulate rumors that he is "dumb" and will not play with him. Acceptance of the child as he is, for better or for worse, is of cardinal importance for any child. This feeling of belonging, or the lack of it, is communicated to the child early in life, even when complete deafness is present.

THE IMPORTANCE OF EARLY DISCOVERY

It is an unfortunate fact that the deaf adults of today were, in all probability, once deaf or hard of hearing children. With early discovery this handicap might have been prevented or made less severe. Frequently the hearing loss increases as a result of neglect or improper care. The situation is further complicated when the child enters school, since his educational growth may lag as much as two or three years behind the other children of his age. At that time he develops psychologic barriers which may prevent normal associations with other children.[15]

Once a child is in school his hearing handicap is relatively easy to identify. Most severely deaf children have been located before they are six years old. However, the partially deaf may go undetected through infancy, early childhood and on into school. Reduced audition in these children is reflected in the failure of the child to respond to loud sounds, defective or delayed speech, social immaturity, unusual behavior patterns, educational or supposed mental retardation.

Ideally, hearing loss should be discovered during the child's first year of life. Developing an awareness of the symptoms in those who have contact with the child and his parents is basic in early case finding. The physician who routinely checks the baby's development, the public health nurse who sees him at intervals in well child conferences or during a visit to his home, the leader of a child study group in which the parents participate and the parents themselves must all be alerted to the symptoms of deafness. One unusually observant mother, Mrs. Spencer Tracy, relates her experience as follows:

When our son, Johnny, was about ten months old he was taking a nap out on the sleeping porch. I decided to wake him as it was about four o'clock. I started out to the sleeping porch and I suppose I was humming along, as mothers do, saying something about it being time to wake up now. I remember very distinctly that I slammed the screen door—you remember things like that sometimes. Yes, I slammed the screen door after me. Still Johnny didn't wake up. I stopped beside his crib. I said, "Johnny, time to wake up," and I saw he wasn't waking. I went still closer and said it again and again until I fairly shouted in his ear, "Johnny, wake up!" Then finally, very gently, I touched him. His eyes flew open and he looked up at me. I knew he was deaf.

THE IMPORTANCE OF OTOLOGIC EVALUATION

Hearing loss is primarily a medical problem. The diagnosis and treatment of hearing disorders falls within the area of the otorhinolaryngologist, usually referred to as otologist. While it is not always possible to measure the degree of loss in preschool children, the otologist by examination will be able to evaluate the child's hearing mechanism. The results of the examination, along with a detailed account of such etiologic factors as the prenatal, birth and postnatal history, and any hereditary deafness provide the otologist with the basis for making his diagnosis. Treatment or surgery may bring improved hearing in some instances, or will prevent further loss. Where there is no treatment or where hearing is still below normal upon completion of treatment, the program of parent-child training should begin.

THE IMPORTANCE OF EDUCATION

It is evident that the child, the parents and the community must be educated, and it is evident that no one individual or school can accomplish this task alone. The handicap of deafness is largely a language handicap, and the child, because he cannot communicate orally, is denied the richly satisfying ability of sharing his feelings and experiences with others, and of learning from the world around him. Education for the deaf and hard of hearing children, as for normal children, must be aimed at guiding each child into the maximum development of his potentialities. For the deaf and hard of hearing this first necessitates the development of oral communicative skills.   With the auditory sense impaired to some degree, the visual, kinesthetic and tactile senses and whatever residual hearing is present must be utilized as a substitute for the acoustic loss to give the child communicative ability. Communication, as continuous in growth within the child as such physical factors as height and weight, is perhaps the most important avenue in the development of the child to his fullest potential.

REFERENCES

1. MYKLEBUST, HELMER R. AND BRUTTEN, MILTON: A study of the visual perception of deaf children. Acta oto-larying (suppl. 105), 1953.

2. BRILL, T.: Mental hygiene and the deaf. Am. Ann. Deaf 79:279–85, 1934.

3. MYKLEBUST, HELMER R.: Toward a new understanding of the deaf child. Keynote Address, convention of American Instructors of the Deaf, Vancouver, Washington, June 28, 1953.

4. TRACY, MRS. SPENCER: The Role of the Parents in the Education of Young Deaf Children. Address given before the Conference for Parents of Preschool Age Deaf Children, Seattle, September 5, 1953.

5. LASSMAN, GRACE HARRIS: Language for the Preschool Deaf Child. New York, Grune & Stratton, 1950.

6. HEDGECOCK, LeRoy D.: Counselling the parents of acoustically handicapped children. Tr. Am. Acad. Ophth. (Jan.–Feb.), 1952.

7. HEIDER, GRACE M.: Adjustment problems of the deaf child. Nerv. Child 7:38–44, January, 1948.

8. GESELL, ARNOLD: Normal and deaf children in the preschool years. Volta Review 48:632–36, November, 1946.

9. HEIDER, GRACE M. AND HEIDER, FRITZ: Studies of preschool deaf children. Volta Review, May, 1943.

10. PINTER, RUDOLF: A mental survey of the deaf. Journal of Educational Research, XIX, 1928.

11. MYKLEBUST, HELMER R. AND BURCHARD, E. G. L.: A study of the effects of congenital and adventitious deafness on intelligence, personality and social maturity of school children. Journal of Educational Psychology, 36:321–43, 1945.

12. Kirk, Samuel and Streng, Alice: The social competence of deaf and hard of hearing children in a public day school. Am. Ann. Deaf 83:244–54, May, 1938.

13. Springer, N. N.: A comparative study of intelligence of a group of deaf and hearing children. Am. Ann. Deaf 83:138–52, 1938.

14. Myklebust, Helmer R.: Clinical psychology and children with impaired hearing. Volta Review, February, 1948.

15. Landis, James E.: A report on the hearing survey in the public schools of Pennsylvania. Tr. Am. Acad. Ophth. (Jan.–Feb.), 1952.

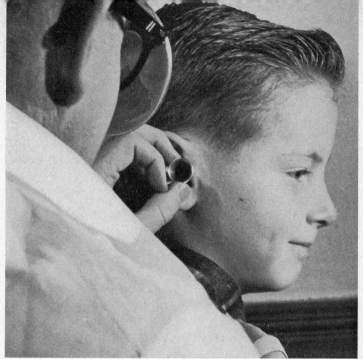

2

Causes of Hearing Losses
and Their Medical Treatment

A QUESTION usually asked first when a child's hearing defect is discovered is "What caused this hearing loss and can it be cured?" Answers naturally vary with the nature of the case, but it is important that parents and teachers be familiar in at least a general way with the causes and medical treatment of hearing disorders.

The interchange of information between the otologist and parents and teachers is essential in helping the acoustically handicapped child. Not the least reason for this is the fact that the parent or teacher who has such information as the physician can supply is in a better position to understand fully the problems faced by the child, and to develop an attitude of accepting the child *as he is* on the basis of this understanding. Too often the parents are unable to develop such an attitude of acceptance, with the result that their emotional attitudes toward the child are unwholesome. Because the problem is not faced realistically, based on an understanding of what can and what cannot be done medically to correct the hearing loss, no really constructive program for the youngster's medical treatment and educational training is planned and put into operation.

Somewhat more obvious is the fact that educational planning for the acoustically handicapped child will be influenced directly by the medical prognosis and by the nature of the disorder. For example, hearing losses which can be improved by medical treatment clearly call for a different type of educational management than do the permanent losses; progressive hearing disabilities present new and important factors which must govern the type of training the child receives. The type of hearing loss sometimes has specialized educational implications in deciding such questions as whether or not to use a hearing aid or other amplification. Equally obvious is the need for the teacher to be constantly alert to symptoms in the child which call for medical attention, and to see that such a referral is carried through by the parents.

The following section presents a discussion of the common causes of hearing loss in children and an explanation of the medical treatment which is available for their correction. First, however, a brief description of the mechanism of hearing will be necessary, since an understanding of hearing defects must rest on some knowledge of the anatomy and physiology of the auditory system.

THE MECHANISM OF THE EAR

From the standpoint of function the process of "hearing" consists basically of a change of sound waves into nerve impulses which reach the brain by way of the auditory nerve and are there interpreted as meaningful sounds. The mechanical conducting system consists of the outer and middle ears which carry the sound energy from the air into the inner ear. At this point the endings of the auditory nerve are stimulated in a certain specialized way by the mechanical energy so that a train of nerve impulses passes along the nerve to certain parts of the brain, which functions in a complex manner to permit us to become aware of a sound and attach an appropriate meaning to it. These structures and their function will be described in more detail in later paragraphs.

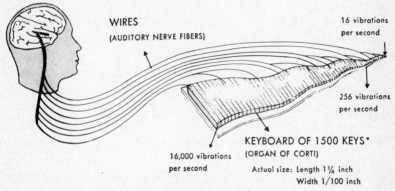

WIRES
(AUDITORY NERVE FIBERS)

16 vibrations
per second

256 vibrations
per second

KEYBOARD OF 1500 KEYS*
(ORGAN OF CORTI)

16,000 vibrations
per second

Actual size: Length 1 ¼ inch
Width 1/100 inch

The hearing mechanism is diagrammatically pictured here. It operates in a manner similar to a piano keyboard—of 1500 keys. Each key responds to the pressure of tones of a particular frequency and to no others, and produces a sound whose pitch differs from that of any other key on the board. The keys are arranged in such a manner that the end key is closed by tones whose frequency is 16 vibrations (double vibrations, d.v., or cycles per second, c.p.s.) per second (the lowest frequency the human ear can hear) and gives rise to the lowest pitch that humans sense. The next key is closed by tones of a slightly higher frequency and gives rise to a slightly higher pitch than the first—and so on down the line, with the last key at the other end of the board receiving tones of a frequency of 16,000 vibrations per second and giving rise to the shrillest of all sounds. (Illustration courtesy Doho Chemical Corporation.)

Before attempting a more exact explanation of the auditory system, a few simple facts about sound waves must be given. Sound, insofar as its physical characteristics are concerned, is a form of wave motion. Sound waves often are compared to water waves which follow dropping a pebble in a quiet pool. This simile is, however, more convenient than accurate. All sub-stances which conduct sound are composed of molecules—whether the conducting medium be air, metal or anything else. Unlike a water wave, which consists of up and down movements of the molecules of the fluid, a sound wave consists of a squeezing together or compression of the molecules followed by a "spreading apart" or period of rarefaction as the molecules rebound. It is more accurate to compare sound waves with the vibrations felt in one end of a steel bar when the other end is tapped than to liken them to water movements.

Certain characteristics of sound waves determine what we experience when a sound is heard. The first of these is *frequency,* which gives rise to the subjective perception of the *pitch* of the sound. Bearing in mind that the source of any sound is a vibrating mass of some sort—the vocal folds, a piano string, a mass of air or whatever it may be—the frequency of the sound can be understood simply as the number of vibrations per second. When a pendulum is at rest and is then set into motion it will first move a given distance in one direction, then swing back in the opposite direction, pass through its original point of rest until it has reached its maximum arc and then return once more to the point from which it started; this process will then continue until the energy imparted by the "push" is used up. A complete single pendular movement back and forth represents a *double vibration* (d.v.) which is one of the units employed for measuring the frequency of sound wave. From another point of view the pendulum passes through one complete *cycle* when it has gone through a double vibration, and frequency may therefore be expressed also in terms of cycles per second (c.p.s.).

What we familiarly term *pitch* is a sensation; it is the "highness" or "lowness" of a musical note and is directly related to the frequency of the sound. On the conventional musical scale the pitch of middle C (C_1) has a frequency of 256 c.p.s. The frequency becomes doubled for each succeeding octave. The ear normally is responsive to quite a wide band of frequencies, hence the person with average hearing experiences a range of pitches from very low to very high. Different investigators report varying figures for the normal frequency response of the human ear, but the usual figures quoted are from approximately 16 c.p.s. to 20,000 c.p.s. How wide a frequency range is needed for the best hearing for speech involves a number of variable factors, but for *optimum* speech reception one's hearing should be normal from about 100 c.p.s. to 8,000 c.p.s. Efficient speech reception is possible if one can hear within a more limited frequency range, however, and some of the factors which are of practical importance in this connection will be discussed in a later section.

The foregoing facts about frequency should be held in mind, because a characteristic of certain types of hearing defect is a limitation of the ability to hear certain frequency bands (often the high frequencies) while the acuity for other frequency bands is relatively unimpaired. Such a finding not only contributes to the medical diagnosis, but also governs many aspects of educational planning.

A second important aspect of sound is its *intensity*, a physical phenomenon which governs the *loudness* one experiences when a sound is heard. If we recall the remarks about the swinging pendulum it can easily be seen that the pendulum will swing from its point of rest a distance which depends on the strength of the push. This distance is the *amplitude* of the wave; when a sound wave is graphically represented in the conventional way its amplitude is the distance between the point of rest and the peak of the wave. The intensity of a sound may be thought of as the amount of energy it contains for delivery to the ear per second. This usually is measured in dynes (a unit of force) per square centimeter. The loudness of a sound is obviously related to the amount of sound energy which reaches the ear. It is easy to see, therefore, that the intensity or energy of a sound depends on the amplitude of each wave and on the number of times per second each wave arrives at the ear. The formula for expressing this relationship is *intensity* equals *amplitude*^{2} times *frequency*^{2}. The fact that amplitude and frequency are squared need not trouble the reader who does not grasp its significance, provided he understands that intensity (amount of energy) depends on frequency and amplitude.

In considering defects of hearing we are most directly interested in the *loudness* with which sounds are experienced. When auditory acuity is reduced the ear is less able for some reason to make use of the energy of ordinary sounds in the environment; a sound of a given intensity is less loud to the defective ear than to the normal ear. The lower threshold of hearing is the point at which a sound has just enough energy to give rise to a sensation. The amount of energy in a sound at threshold will vary with the frequency of the sound. These various threshold values have been determined statistically after measurements of large numbers of normal ears and form the basis for testing a child's hearing with the audiometer.

Thus, when we say a child has a hearing loss of a certain amount we mean that in order for him to sense the sound its intensity must be increased beyond what would be necessary for the normal child. The amount of this increase is measured in units called decibels (db) which express amounts of *increase* of intensity of one sound as compared to another. Since measurements must have a starting point, the normal threshold of hearing is assigned the value of zero. When one is told that a child has a 20 decibel loss this means that a sound must, to reach his threshold, have a 20 db greater intensity than would be necessary for its perception by the normal ear.

The mechanism of hearing is ordinarily said to consist of the outer, middle and inner ears. The outer ear includes the auricle and the external auditory canal. The auricle serves primarily to collect sound waves which then pass into the ear canal which runs for a distance of about 25 mm. through the external portion of the temporal bone of the skull. At the inner end of the canal is the tympanum, or ear drum, which separates the outer and middle ears. The cavity of the middle ear contains three small bones—the ossicles—and is connected to the upper part of the throat (nasopharynx) by a canal called the eustachian tube.

The ossicles consist of the malleus, which is attached to the tympanum, the incus, which is articulated with the malleus at one end and with another bone, the stapes, at the other end. The stapes, which is thus the innermost member of this chain of three bones, rests on the partition which separates the middle

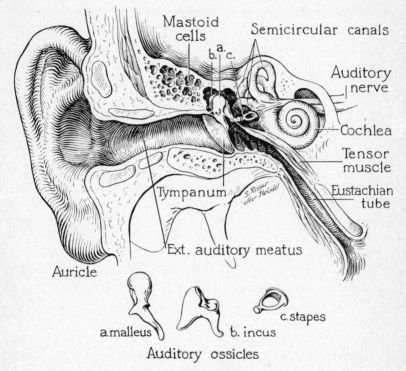

Diagram of the auditory system

ear from the inner ear. This wall is primarily a bony partition, but contains two small membranous windows, on one of which, the oval window (fenestra ovalis), the footplate of the stapes pushes when set in movement. The eustachian tube provides drainage for the middle ear cavity and also allows air to enter so that pressures on either side of the tympanum can be equalized.

The outer and middle ears function as a mechanical conducting system for sound waves. As the sound wave strikes the ear drum, this membrane moves inward and outward in response to the alternating positive and negative pressures of the sound waves (areas of compression and rarefaction). These movements are imparted to the ossicular chain with a resulting somewhat piston-like action of the stapes on the membranous oval window, on the inner side of which is the fluid of the inner ear. This fluid is thus set into motion also. While the basic functioning of this conducting system can be visualized in this simple manner, the middle ear is actually a complex and highly specialized system which not only protects the ear against very strong sound pressures, but also provides efficient transmission for a wide range of sound intensities. Diseases and abnormalities of the outer and middle ear, particularly the latter, cause a hearing loss in a significant number of children.

The inner ear is exceedingly complex and has two principal functions: hearing and the maintenance of posture and equilibrium. The latter depends on the vestibular apparatus and the semicircular canals, which need not be discussed here although their presence near the end organ of hearing explains why, in some types of disease, symptoms such as dizziness (vertigo) and loss of equilibrium may be associated with a hearing defect. Hearing is mediated by the cochlear portion of the inner ear which contains the terminal fibers of the acoustic branch of the VIIIth cranial nerve (auditory nerve).

The cochlea is a cone-shaped tube which winds spirally two and three-quarters times, giving it the external appearance of a snail shell. If a cross section of the tube were made at any point one could observe that the canal is bisected by a partition consisting of a narrow bony shelf (osseus spiral lamina) projecting from the side nearest the inner core of the cochlea (modiolus) and a membrane, the basilar membrane, which runs from the spiral lamina to the outer wall of the tube. The portion of the tube below the basilar membrane is the scala tympani and contains a fluid, perilymph. The upper half of the tube is further divided into two approximately equal parts by another membrane, Reissner's membrane, which runs laterally upward and outward from the spiral lamina to the outer wall of the tube at an angle of about 45°. The canal above Reissner's membrane is the scala vestibuli and the one between it and the basilar membrane is the scala media or cochlear duct. Both are filled with lymph fluid. At the very tip of the spirally wound cochlea is a small opening (helicotrema) between the scala vestibuli and the scala tympani. On the basilar membrane throughout its length is a cluster of specialized cells called the Organ of Corti within which are the nerve endings which transmit the impulses leading to a sensation of hearing.

The arrangement of these canals is such that when movements of the stapes occur vibrations of the fluid in the vestibule pass onward to the scala vestibuli around the turns of the cochlea and through the helicotrema to the fluid within the scala tympani, thus passing on either side of the basilar membrane. At the termination of the scala tympani is a second membranous window (fenestra rotunda) which presumably facilitates movement of the cochlear fluid. Anatomically, the round window is located near the oval window on the bony partition between the middle and inner ears.

The exact way in which these vibrations in the fluid are transformed into nerve impulses is not completely understood and a number of differing theoretic explanations have been offered. Presumably the movements of the basilar membrane itself and of the Organ of Corti which reflect the vibrations of the fluid play an important role. Nevertheless, it is clear that the translation of mechanical movements into nerve impulses takes place within the cochlea.

Nerve impulses thus aroused are propagated along the cochlear branch of the VIIIth cranial nerve to the temporal lobe of the brain, and from this point to other areas of the cortex by means of complex networks of nerve fibers (neurones). The general term *perceptive loss* is sometimes used to describe any defect of hearing caused by failure of this neural transmitting system. It is probably less confusing, however, to use the term *nerve loss* and to confine this type of hearing defect to a break-

down of the neural mechanisms in the cochlea or along the
course of the cochlear nerve to a point just before its fibers end
in the layers of the cerebral cortex in the temporal lobe of the
brain.

The role of the brain itself in hearing is very important, of
course, but involves a basically different kind of function than
that of the peripheral hearing mechanism which has been described in the foregoing paragraphs. All that reaches the brain
is a series of nerve impulses which in themselves are without
meaning. What the brain does, however, is to sort these nerve
impulses out, interpret and attach meaning to them and direct
the results of this *perception* to other parts of the brain where
they may be used in a way which is useful to the organism. It is
entirely possible, for instance, for an individual to be aware of
speech, in the sense that his hearing mechanism operates normally, but be unable to understand what is heard because the
brain does not function as it should. The latter defect should
not be thought of as a hearing loss, however, but as a breakdown
in the higher functions of the brain itself.

In children who are brain injured there may be defects of
speech and language which resemble those associated with hearing loss, and the child's behavior may be like that of a hard of
hearing or deaf youngster. Often it is quite difficult clinically to
distinguish between a purely sensory loss and a breakdown of
the higher brain functions, particularly with younger children,
and mistaken diagnoses are sometimes made. Such terms as
"word deafness," "central deafness" and the like are sometimes
employed to describe disorders involving brain function, but the
use of the word "deafness" in this connection is misleading. In
general, these disorders fall into the category of *aphasia,* which
may be defined as a defect of language, or appear as a form of
auditory *agnosia,* which is a loss of comprehension of auditory
sensations. Other perceptual difficulties of the brain injured
child may also interfere with language development and thus
create a suspicion of hearing loss where there is no real sensory
defect. Obviously these various possibilities must be taken into

account in studying the child who is thought to have an auditory handicap.

Diseases of the Ear

With the foregoing discussion of certain aspects of sound as they relate to hearing it is now possible to turn to an explanation of the types of hearing loss and the most commonly encountered diseases which cause reduced hearing. It will naturally not be possible to give a detailed presentation of each disease, nor does space permit mention of the rarer pathologic conditions. An effort will be made, however, to include the essential facts concerning the various diseases in order that the nonmedical therapist and parent may interpret the child's problem intelligently. One should bear in mind, of course, that methods of treatment constantly undergo change and improvement and that all children with hearing loss should be under continuing medical supervision.

Hearing losses may be classified into two types: (1) obstructive (conduction) losses and (2) nerve (perception) losses. The term obstructive loss refers to a rise in the auditory threshold through interference with the function of the mechanical conducting system of the ear. Diseases causing obstructive losses therefore attack either the outer or middle ears in such a way that sound vibrations are not carried through to the fluid of the inner ear in the manner described earlier. Nerve losses occur when the cochlear branch of the auditory nerve does not conduct the appropriate impulses (aroused originally by movements of the cochlear fluid) to the brain itself. The disorder therefore involves either the basilar membrane or Organ of Corti (or both) in the cochlea or else limits or abolishes the conducting capacity of the nerve somewhere along its course. Mixed hearing losses, including both obstructive and nerve defect, are common although one of the two elements always predominates.

The differentiation and relative effects of these two types of auditory defect is possible with a high degree of accuracy through combined otologic examination and audiometric measurement. If the air conduction audiogram, a chart of the auditory threshold at certain low, middle and high pitches made by use of an earphone placed on the ear, shows that the child does not hear normally the physician knows only that a loss exists; he cannot say with certainty whether the condition is one of obstructive, nerve or mixed type, although the pattern of the loss at each of the frequencies may be strongly suggestive. A second method of testing, based on *bone conduction,* may be used: this employs a special type of receiver placed firmly against the bone behind the ear in such a way that the sound vibrations are lead to the fluid of the inner ear through the temporal bone, rather than by the usual channel. Bone conduction and air conduction graphs are then compared. If the child hears normally by bone conduction, but not by air conduction, one assumes that the nerve is functioning normally since it obviously is responding to stimulation. In this case the diagnosis is one of obstructive loss and the defect is to be found in either the outer or middle ear. If, on the other hand, bone conduction hearing is no better than the air conduction threshold the otologist must conclude that the auditory nerve is not functioning, since it appears unable to respond to stimulation no matter how the vibrations are led to the inner ear fluid. There are various specialized tests giving more detailed information about the type and extent of loss and the relative function of each ear, but all depend basically on the foregoing principle. The results of the hearing test therefore give the otologist clues as to where to look for a diseased condition.

The Causes of Obstructive Losses

Congenital Defects

One of the most difficult problems is that of abnormalities of development of the auricle and external ear canals. Embryologically, the development of the ossicles, the auditory nerve endings, the auditory canal and auricle is a complicated process, and numerous anomalies may be found when there has been an interruption in their formation. While this may occur on one side only, it is more commonly bilateral. The auricle may be represented by a single tab of skin, or perhaps several unrelated nodules of tissue without any cartilage support. Of more serious nature, the external ear canal may be narrowed or may end in a blind pouch a few millimeters below the skin surface. X-rays show no bony canals, although the mastoid antrum and mastoid cells may be identified. Fusion of the malleus and incus is a common occurrence. There may be cochlear abnormalities which result in defects of auditory perception.

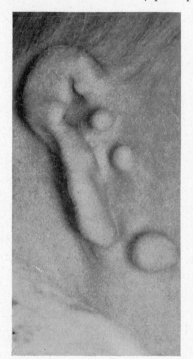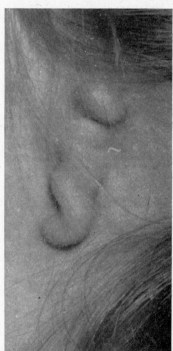

Congenital malformation of the auricle (microtia) with absence of the external ear canal.

In complete absence of the ear canal there is about a 50 db hearing loss. Accurate determination is difficult, but estimations by speech and conditioned reflex tests may be made in the young child. Later, audiometry gives an accurate picture of the true loss.

The only practical way to improve hearing is the surgical creation of a serviceable ear canal. Due to the mechanical difficulty of working with small structure, it is best to delay such procedure until the child is from three to nine years old. After creating an epithelial lined tract to the skull behind the mandibular articulation, a hole is made in the bone to the mastoid antrum. If the stapes to cochlear system is uninvolved, hearing will be improved to a 30 db level by this procedure alone. The maleus and incus are identified and removed, for if fused they act to impede the transmission of sound. If the stapes is fixed, little hearing improvement will be noted postoperatively. In such a case a fenestration procedure (see otosclerosis, page 45) may be undertaken. The creation of auricles by means of skin pedicle flaps is usually a long process and falls in the field of plastic surgery. Before undertaking surgical correction, all concerned—the patient, surgeon and audiologist—should have clearly in mind the special goal in each particular case.

External Ear Disease

External otitis is an inflammation of the ear canal caused by bacteria, various types of fungi or eczema-like skin conditions. It is found throughout the United States but is most prevalent in subtropical areas. It is particularly associated with moisture, as around swimming areas, and is noted for its chronicity and tendency to reoccurrence. In the acute stage there is severe swelling of the canal walls until the lumen is obliterated. If the infection is limited to a hair follicle or sebaceous gland it is called a circumscribed otitis externa, or furunculosis. The swelling may be so great and the pain so intense that acute mastoiditis is simulated. A diffuse external canal infection is one in which the involvement was spread throughout the canal circumference. Pain is severe and there is considerable swelling. At the same time, there is severe itching, and a thin watery discharge which in a few days changes to a cheesy desquamated material. Tenderness of the neck and swollen lymph glands are usual complications.

The chronic stage is characterized by long-standing inflammation and discharge with crusting, reddened and cracked skin around the orifice and ear lobe. Cultures and sensitivity tests of the discharge are required to determine the causative organism, and to aid in the treatment. Frequent secondary factors are numerous pathogenic and nonpathogenic fungi. An eczema may also develop with an intense itching and skin irritation which may result in an actual stenosis, or closure of the canal. While not painful the condition causes an annoyance and irritation from the discharge.

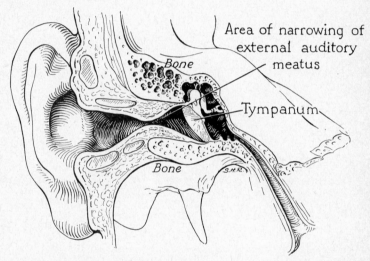

Stenosis of the External Ear Canal. Stenosis is a partial occlusion of the external ear canal; atresia is a complete occlusion. Either condition prevents normal hearing and may be caused by congenital malformation of the soft tissue, bony tissue or both, or by injury or inflammation of the external ear canal.

Treatment in the acute phase consists of sedation and gentle local cleansing with such solutions as urea and cortisone preparations to relieve swelling. After the offending organism is identified the most effective drugs locally, and specific antibiotics systemically may be selected. In the absence of laboratory identification, one of the standard drugs may be selected for trial.

Careful cleansing and the application of wicks or packs saturated in antiseptic solutions several times weekly over a long
period will usually control the disease. Treatment must be continued after symptoms subside to destroy bacteria situated in
the crypts, glands and hair follicles. In severe infections the
wax glands become so depressed or destroyed that no wax is
formed for periods up to several months. Since this material is
important in the prevention of infection, a substitute to prevent
dryness and scaling should be introduced. There is ordinarily
no permanent damage to the ear drum or ear canal, and hearing
will return to its pre-inflammation level when the swelling subsides and the drainage stops.

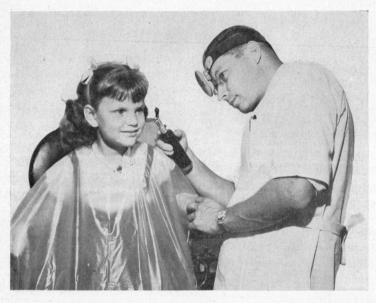

The otoscope is used to visualize the external auditory canal and the
drum membrane. (Photo courtesy Washington State Department of Health)

Foreign bodies which obstruct the external auditory meatus
constitute a frequent cause of hearing loss. By far the most common foreign body is ear wax (cerumen), a substance secreted by

glands of the external ear canal and present to some extent in everyone. For some unknown reason, some individuals produce a great deal of wax which, if not removed, may harden into a plug which blocks the ear canal. This condition is not considered a disease, nor does it appear to be associated with excessive activity of glands of a similar nature in other parts of the body.

There is no successful treatment for excessive secretion of wax, but periodic removal of obstructions is a relatively simple process when undertaken by a physician. Parents, however, are cautioned against attempting the procedure unless they are acting under instructions from the doctor. Most often wax is removed by irrigation of the external ear canal with water, although at times it may be necessary to loosen or soften the impacted cerumen with oily solutions. Small instruments may also be used to get at the wax. Other types of foreign bodies which may find their way into the ear canal—beans, cotton, chewing gum, rubber erasers and other small miscellaneous objects—may be flushed out by irrigation or may require removal by a hook-like instrument which is used to dislodge the obstruction.

Middle Ear Disease

Secretory otitis is a term used to describe the condition in which there is a collection of fluid of varying consistency in the middle ear. It is similar to what has been called nonsuppurative catarrhal otitis, since the material is sterile for both bacteria and virus infection. It is not therefore primarily an infection but a static collection of fluid. It results from a closure of the eustachian tube, and may be due to lymphoid tissue at the tubal orifice, nasal or sinus disease or allergy. Rapid changes in altitude in air travel and attenuated otitis media caused by the widespread use of antibiotics have made this disease more common in late years.

The usual symptoms are deafness, fullness of the ear and autophony. There may be slight pain or occasional dizziness. On physical examination the eardrum appears abnormal but the changes are frequently slight. There is an oil-paper appearance of the drum, and through it may be seen a fluid level and enclosed air bubbles. Hearing loss is no greater than 30 db. If the eustachian tube is inflated, bubbly sounds may be heard. There are no systemic symptoms and the nose and throat examination may be quite normal.

Treatment by tubal inflation is occasionally successful early, but is ineffective if the fluid is partially solidified. The most simple technique is that of needle puncture of the drum and aspiration. In cases of long duration, and this may persist over a period of years, the fluid is mucoid or jelly-like and other methods must be used. The drum is incised and spot suction used, possibly with simultaneous eustachian tube inflation. In cases where some of the mastoid cells are filled, large amounts of material are removed. These procedures, if undertaken on children, should be done under general anesthesia, as they may be painful and tedious and must be done carefully.

Otitis media, an infective condition of the middle ear, is by far the most frequent condition causing low grade and moderate hearing loss in children, and is thought to be responsible for as much as half of the hearing defects among adults. Middle ear infection may manifest itself in various ways, and may be either chronic or acute. Acute attacks have a sudden onset with severe earache associated with fever and accompanied sometimes by spontaneous rupture of the eardrum with consequent drainage of purulent material from the external ear. More frequently the ear does not drain and the inflammation subsides within a few days, particularly when treatment with one of the new antibiotics is instituted. In a large number of cases the attack of otitis media is not recognized as such by the parent, even though the child may complain of an earache.

Otitis media results from infection through invasion of the middle ear by pathogenic bacteria which ordinarily ascend through the eustachian tube. Thus, middle ear infections may be associated with any type of upper respiratory tract infection, sinusitis, or may be an important sequel to a number of children's diseases such as measles and chicken pox. Isolated attacks of otitis media, particularly where medical treatment of the infection is begun promptly, ordinarily do not result in any permanent loss of hearing, although there may be exceptions to this generalization. Chronic otitis media, on the other hand, is a very grave threat to hearing.

Damage to the mechanism of the middle ear may occur in various ways. Repeated or chronic inflammation is likely to produce very fine adhesions between the eardrum and the bones of the middle ear and between the ossicles themselves. Adhesions also form at the opening of the eustachian tube. Such adhesions involving the ossicles and eardrum prevent the normal transmission of sound waves. If this fibrotic and scarring process has been repeated many times over a long period of time the ossicles and the oval and round windows may become so matted down that there is no hope of their regaining normal mobility. The eardrum may also be involved as a consequence of a kind of decay (*necrosis*) which sets in when otitis media is chronic, with the result that the tympanum may become perforated, and subsequently scarred and thickened. Rupture of the drum in an acute attack will cause scarring also, although a hearing loss may not follow. Perforation of the drum, in addition to its possible effect on hearing, is also a potentially dangerous condition for the patient since there is an open pathway for the entrance of bacteria into the middle ear.

Mastoiditis represents a more serious complication of middle ear disease. This occurs when the infection extends from the middle ear cavity backward into the mastoid bone. An acute mastoiditis may flare up in the same way that acute otitis media does, but mastoiditis which follows chronic otitis media is much more common. A severe hearing loss may usually be expected. Symptoms to be watched for include a slowly progressive hearing loss which may be detected by hearing tests repeated at regular intervals. A more dramatic warning signal may be the occurrence of repeated attacks of earache with or without a draining ear. The ear discharge is, of course, a major symptom in itself. Treatment of mastoiditis is initiated by the vigorous and continuing use of antibiotics and other measures by which the otologist often controls the inflammation. If these measures fail, he must turn to surgery to "clean up" the infection. Fortunately, such operations, once very common, have now been made unnecessary in many cases because of the development of new antibiotic drugs.

Mastoidectomy may be either simple or radical. In the simple mastoidectomy only the diseased bone is removed, without disturbing the structures in the middle ear. This may leave the hearing relatively good or even normal in favorable cases. A radical mastoidectomy, however, involves removal not only of the diseased bone but also of the structures of the middle ear and necrotic portions of the walls of the middle ear cavity. This will always cause a more severe hearing loss, since both eardrum and ossicles are removed.

Obviously the most important consideration is prevention of mastoiditis and other consequences of chronic otitis media through prompt and thorough treatment of middle ear infection. To the otologist, the manner in which parents neglect symptoms of ear disease and the home remedies employed for their relief are a continuing source of amazement. Even a simple earache with no other apparent symptoms should be reported to the doctor. A discharging ear demands immediate medical treatment, while repeated attacks of otitis media—often occurring in the winter months—call for conscientious and continued treatment of a type in which the thoughtless parent sometimes does not cooperate. The otologist will first undertake to control the inflammation itself and, in the case of chronic disease, will go on to search for and correct the causes of the repeated attacks. These causes will be those nose and throat conditions which are the source of the bacterial invasion of the eustachian tube and middle ear. By far the most common cause in childhood is hypertrophied (enlarged) and infected tonsils and adenoids. The eustachian tube opens within a few millimeters of both tonsils and adenoids, and an inflammation within these two units of lymph tissue is responsible for perhaps 75 per cent of the ear trouble in children. A second condition which is often responsible for middle ear disease is nasal and sinus infection. If an infected sinus persistently discharges a purulent secretion over either one or both of the eustachian tube openings there will undoubtedly be inflammatory changes within the ears.

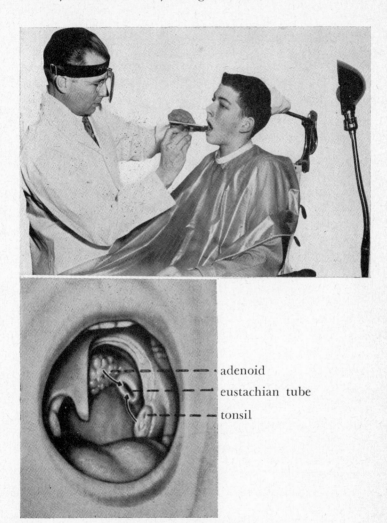

adenoid
eustachian tube
tonsil

Light reflected in the tiny magnifying mirror placed in the back of the mouth is used to visualize the nasopharynx, tonsils, adenoids and eustachian tube orifices. (Photo courtesy Washington State Department of Health; diagram courtesy Doho Chemical Corporation)

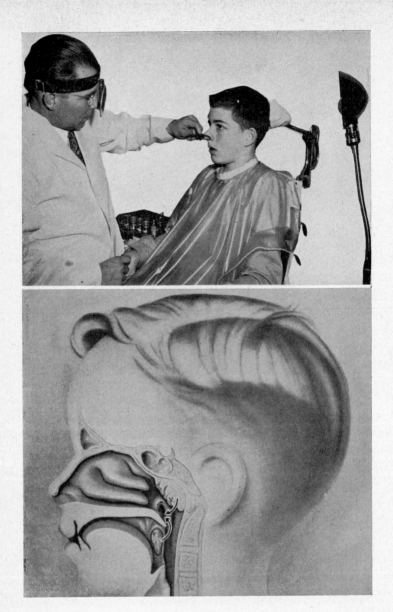

The nasal speculum is used to visualize the nasal mucous membranes, turbinates and septum. (Photo courtesy Washington State Department of Health; diagram courtesy Doho Chemical Corporation)

Injury to the eardrum and parts of the middle ear leading to hearing loss is fortunately not particularly common, but such accidents may occur. Perforation of the eardrum by an object thrust into the ear canal is perhaps the most frequent mishap. In such a case the ossicular chain may also be damaged. Head injuries, particularly those involving basal skull fractures, occasionally involve middle ear damage, and may also cause nerve destruction. The effects of blasts or extremely loud noises on the middle ear are well known, but children are not ordinarily placed in circumstances where they suffer hearing loss as a consequence of such conditions. It is conceivable that a "slap" on the ear might drive air into the external ear canal with sufficient force to rupture the eardrum, although this must certainly be a rare occurrence. Perforations of the drum can sometimes be closed by mechanical devices or by skin grafts. Recently, procedures to reconstruct the eardrum and diseased ossicles have been developed. The damaged drum and bones are replaced by a skin graft which vibrates like a new eardrum. These operations, myringoplasty and tympanoplasty, not only seal the middle ear from outside infection, but often improve hearing to a serviceable level.

Otosclerosis, while not primarily a disease of young children, merits discussion because it is reported to have been detected as early as the seventh year. The wide publicity that has been given to the fenestration operation for the improvement of hearing in otosclerosis also makes it important for the parent and teacher to understand that such surgery is successful only for losses caused by this disease, and even then only in certain carefully selected cases.

Otosclerosis, or hardening of the inner ear bone, involves the region where the stapes joins the inner ear mechanism. Although present at birth, it often does not produce noticeable hearing loss until later in life, usually after the age of twenty. As the bony hardening continues, it involves the inner ear itself, causing deterioration of the hearing nerve. Therefore a mixed type of hearing impairment is found, with increased involvement in the higher frequencies.

The cause of otosclerosis is unknown: It has been found to occur more often in females, and pregnancy seems to aggravate the process in some instances. Although often hereditary, increasing consideration is being given to the possibility that vascular and metabolic factors are of importance.

The principal symptom of otosclerosis is a gradual loss of hearing in both ears, without evidence of associated systemic infection or specific ear infection. When x-rays are taken the temporal bones will typically show no evidence of residual infection. The eardrums will be normal in appearance. In most cases the hearing loss has its onset after puberty, although cases of earlier onset have been described in the literature. Many cases of otosclerosis do not come to the attention of the otologist until late in the victim's 'teens or in his early twenties. Head noises (tinnitus) are present, or may have been present at some time in the past. The hearing loss may have been slowly progressive for a time, then apparently stationary, or it may have been steadily progressive. In typical otosclerosis air conduction thresholds are approximately 30 db or more above (or worse than) bone conduction thresholds, demonstrating that the defect is in the middle ear. Blood relatives of the same or antecedent generations usually either have or have had a similar complaint.

Otosclerosis is not benefited by local or medical treatment. Surgical procedures for restoration of hearing date back to the late 19th century, but were not regarded as offering good promise of success until improvement of technique was devised by American surgeons. Today, with the advent of electronic equipment to test hearing, adequate illumination and magnification and modern drugs to combat infection, two types of operations are widespread.

Stapes mobilization is performed under local anesthesia. The ear drum is carefully elevated to expose the stapes which is deliberately manipulated until it loosens and is movable. The ear drum is then replaced in its normal position. The patient may be hospitalized only a few days. If the procedure is successful the patient gains much with little inconvenience. In selected cases approximately 60 per cent of patients regain serviceable hearing.

Fenestration is carried out under general anesthesia. The principle of the operation is basically the creation of a small window, the size of a grain of rice, in the inner ear (horizontal semicircular canal). A skin flap is laid over the newly created window. The ear drum is intact but the ossicular chain is separated. The principle involved is the creation of a new pathway through which sound pressures may bypass the fixed stapes area and stimulate the auditory nerve. The patient is hospitalized a week, and is away from his activities for an additional two or three weeks. In 80 per cent of the cases suitable for fenestration, hearing can be restored to a serviceable level. There are various sources of failure for the operation, but the chief ones are regrowth of bone across the window and failure to select only patients whose auditory nerves can function adequately when they are once more subject to stimulation. The techniques of selection of subjects and surgery are both undergoing constant improvement.

THE CAUSES OF NERVE LOSSES

While the number of children with hearing losses due to nerve involvement is much less than the number with obstructive defects, nerve loss usually presents a more severe degree of hearing handicap—often reaching the degree of total deafness—when it does occur. The general pathology of nerve losses includes (1) hereditary defects of the inner ear and cochlear nerve, (2) disease affecting the fetus in the intrauterine stage and (3) postnatal disease or injury.

Heredity appears to be responsible for a fairly consistent percentage of cases. Such hereditary factors involve the epithelial cells which are destined to form the inner ear. This may take the form of a failure to develop the specialized cells which form the nerve element of the Organ of Corti, or there may be a tendency toward early degeneration of the fundamental cells. The mechanism by which this defect is transmitted in the blood line is the same as that for such things as hair color, facial features and the like. This condition is not a disease in the sense that it involves pathologic tissue change, but is a true agenesis or developmental failure. The presence of deafness in a child's family history is considered very suggestive of possible hereditary loss, but such a defect may occur without known familial deafness. There is no type of therapy for this kind of case, and gross otologic examinations are all negative.

Damage to the hearing apparatus before birth is most often caused by what is called a neurotropic virus, or one having a special affinity for the nervous system. The same virus which affects hearing may also cause other types of nerve damage, including lesions in the higher brain centers of the type which lead to the condition called cerebral palsy. This fact offers a partial explanation for the fact that a substantial percentage of the cerebral palsied youngsters have reduced audition. Of the neurotropic viruses, that of German measles (rubella) is apparently the most frequent offender. The most critical time is from approximately the second to fourth months of fetal life, since this is the period when a greatly accelerated growth of the nervous system, particularly the brain, is taking place. In most instances the mother is known to have been ill, although a definite diagnosis of rubella may not have been made at the time, but it is thought also that the virus may be passed on to the child without any apparent sickness on the part of the mother. Other types of virus infection may also affect the fetal nervous system, but these are less well identified as compared to the rubella virus. It is also felt that spirochetal (syphilitic) involvement of the central nervous system may occur during the early months of pregnancy. Effective control of syphilis in the mother is possible, and modern obstetric practice makes tests for syphilis a matter of routine, so that the frequency of hearing loss from such a cause is becoming negligible. There is some evidence that maternal use of certain drugs such as quinine and salicylic acid (derivatives of which may be used to relieve pain) may affect the fetus. There is a great deal of variation in the individual susceptibility to any of the drugs, and even small doses may cause severe damage in some persons.

Hemorrhage occurring during the process of birth (prenatal period) or shortly after birth (neonatal period) may be responsible for hearing losses. There are, of course, numerous causes for hemorrhage including trauma from prolonged or rapid delivery, caesarian section, breech presentation, other abnormal birth conditions and inept obstetric practice. In addition, another class of causes for bleeding will be such things as oxygen deprivation (anoxia) and blood abnormalities such as that caused by Rh incompatibility, which may be present when certain differences in blood type exist between the parents. The whole subject is much too complex for presentation in a discussion of this type, but the general principle is that any of the conditions which may cause brain damage may involve the neural elements in the hearing mechanism. There is no known medical treatment which will improve hearing in any of the foregoing types of cases, a fact which makes adequate educational provision for these children of the utmost importance. This, in turn, makes early discovery of the loss an urgent matter.

Many infections which cause a hearing defect strike after birth, quite often between the second and seventh years of life. Meningitis and encephalitis are chief offenders, accounting for perhaps 20 per cent of cases of severely nerve deafened children. These diseases are characterized by a kind of scarring of the covering of the brain in such a manner that transmission of nerve impulses is blocked at points which depend on the particular area which becomes involved. Widespread degenerative changes in the neural substance itself, in the brain and cranial nerves (one of which, the VIIIth, functions in hearing), are observed in severe cases. Oddly enough, there seems to be little relation between the severity of infection and the degree to which hearing may be involved. A child who is severely ill with meningitis may recover with no nerve involvement, while another child who seemed much less sick may suffer a severe hearing loss or some other distressing sequel. Vigorous treatment of meningitis with the newer drugs of the penicillin and mycin group has greatly reduced the mortality of this highly fatal disease; and hence, an increased number of cases with hearing loss from this cause is to be anticipated.

Whereas meningitis is an inflammation of the coverings of the brain and spinal cord, encephalitis is a condition in which the brain substance itself is involved. In meningoencephalitis the two may be combined. Encephalitis may be caused by a wide variety of organisms, chiefly viruses, many of which remain unidentified. These inflammations act much as do those in meningitis in their formation of scar tissue which may interrupt the function of one or more of the cranial nerves. In both meningitis and encephalitis there may, of course, be grave effects other than hearing loss, including paralysis, widespread changes in behavior, mental defect and other sensory defects. In some instances several of the so-called children's diseases may terminate in an encephalitis, notably mumps. Meningitis and encephalitis as a result of immunization shots and vaccination are not unknown.

For the most part, any loss of hearing from nerve damage is irreparable insofar as medical treatment is concerned. There is no evidence that the damaged neural elements can regenerate and hence regain function. In an occasional child with a nerve loss, however, some restoration of auditory acuity seems to take place although dramatic and significant improvement should never be hoped for. In those children who seem to get better, it is always difficult to say whether there actually has been a real improvement in hearing or whether the child has learned only to be more responsive to sound and to make a more intelligent use of what he hears. The latter certainly happens with many hard of hearing children who seem to hear more acutely after educational training, but whose thresholds on careful testing prove to be no better than before training started.

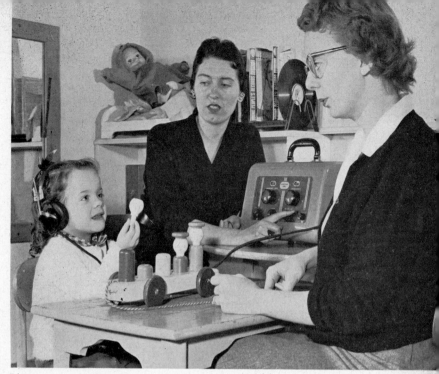

3

Audiometry and Case Finding

CASE finding goes far beyond the narrow concept of merely locating a child who is deaf or hard of hearing. It is concerned with recognizing children who have potential ear trouble or hearing defects, so that the disability can be prevented. Moreover, case finding provides a basis for estimating the extent, distribution and severity of the problem of hearing loss in a community, and is a guide to the need for personnel, services and facilities necessary to carry out a program of prevention and rehabilitation.

The important first step in any program of hearing conservation is to find the individual children who need care or further

study and to bring them to the attention of the appropriate professional person or agency in a position to provide the right
kind of help.[1]

RECOGNITION OF CHILDREN WITH HEARING PROBLEMS

A hearing loss is usually a subtle, "unseen" defect, frequently
unknown to the child himself because he does not know how
well he ought to hear, and sometimes difficult for the observer
to detect. Thus early recognition of the child who has or who
may develop a hearing defect is not always easy. A medical history which inquires into the following areas may give indication
of hearing loss:

> hearing loss in other members of the family;
> complications of pregnancy, delivery, prematurity, neonatal
>   disease;
> acute infections in which the ears may be involved;
> repeated upper respiratory infections, acute otitis, chronic
>   middle ear disease.

Children with these conditions in their backgrounds may be
considered vulnerable and should receive more than routine
follow-up, including hearing tests appropriate to their age.

Parents may not suspect deafness in an infant until the baby
is about a year old. He does not turn toward them when they
speak to him, he fails to react to loud sounds, and his vocalizations remain at the babbling stage, or may gradually cease.
Young children with less severe impairment may attempt
speech, but it is usually delayed or defective.

Hearing loss may be suspected when a child:

> seems more aware of movement than sound;
> responds better when watching the speaker's face, particu
>   larly the lips;
> has a strained expression when listening;
> is inattentive to things which are of interest to children of
>   his age;
> has defective speech or an unusual voice quality;

confuses words which sound alike;

is less socially adequate than children of his age.

Because case finding is a continuous process it should begin early in the preschool years and continue during a child's school experience. All community resources should be explored for help in locating these children. In this connection, certain sources of information are of particular importance:

1. *Parents* who suspect a hearing loss when their child does not develop appropriate speech and language, or does not respond to auditory stimuli like other children.

2. *Public Health Nurses* who see children in schools, health conferences, in a visit to the home or suspect a hearing defect on the basis of family history or other symptoms.

3. *Teachers* who see a child in relation to the other children in the class and may suspect a hearing loss based on school performance or periodic hearing screening.

4. *Physicians* who recognize hearing loss or ear disease on the basis of physical examination, or may suspect it from the family or medical history.

5. *Records in Child Health Clinics, Medical or Guidance Clinics* on preschool children who show unusually slow language development or behavior suggesting a hearing loss.

PERIODIC HEARING SCREENING

Most children with severe hearing losses are located early in life, but a high proportion of those with mild and moderate impairments will be missed without periodic screening tests for children of all ages. Responsibility for these routine examinations of infants and young children rests with the physicians who provide health supervision for these children in their offices or in child health clinics. In some communities routine testing of children, just before their entrance to school, is arranged for by health or education authorities in preschool roundups, clinics or nursery schools.

Various methods may be used to screen hearing acuity and to detect hearing loss. The method selected must be geared to the age group and maturity of the children tested, as well as to the qualifications of the individuals who make the evaluations.

INFANCY TO AGE FOUR

In general, quantitative routine screening tests of hearing for children under four years of age yield only presumptive evidence that hearing may or may not be within normal limits. Qualitative tests for young children are discussed in Chapter 4. In many instances the presumptive evidence of quantitative tests serves to reinforce behavioral evidence, such as the child's responses to everyday sounds. Downs, in a report of a hearing test for preschool children developed by her at the University of Denver, uses recorded familiar sounds including a dog bark, cat meow, car horn, gun shot, telephone bell and bird song. These sounds are presented at known intensity levels. The test is reported to be successful in case finding at the preschool level.

Infants four to six months of age respond best in test situations to the human voice, especially to a familiar, quiet one. The baby will usually turn his head toward the source of sound when spoken to, and will show pleasure on hearing known voices. At six to twelve months the baby with normal hearing recognizes many meaningful sounds, and his own vocalization becomes more varied and specialized.

Between ages one and two, the child with normal hearing understands an increasing number of words and begins to say some. He is learning to vocalize with some accuracy. After two years of age, a normally hearing child may be expected to respond to appropriate suggestions spoken behind his back.

From ages four to six, gross, quantitative test methods are more suitable. The child is not quite ready for the more accurate audiometric measurement which requires his sustained attention and cooperation. Certain crude tests such as watch tick, whisper, spoken voice and tuning fork tests are useful for gross evaluation of hearing. If a child seems to hear a sound only at half the distance at which a normally hearing person can hear it, there may be significant hearing loss. These tests are not standardized and are useful only for an approximate hearing screening where more exact methods cannot be used. In the late preschool period, many children if adequately prepared can be screened accurately with an audiometer.

Hearing Screening for School Children

Hearing loss ranks relatively high in the scale of handicapping conditions that affect school children. Landis, reporting a 1952 hearing survey of approximately 50,000 school children in Pennsylvania, estimates there are one to three children in every classroom with some degree of defective hearing, or from three to four per cent of the school population. Other investigations estimate the incidence at 5 per cent of children under the age of twenty years.[2] Hardy states that for every ten children screened out with hearing or speech-hearing impairment, eight fall into the subclinical or marginal group about which modern otology and medicine in general can do the most. Thus the vast proportion of these children are fully redeemable in terms of the physical disability if the impairment is discovered soon after its onset and if proper medical care is begun. For the two out of ten who have irreversible hearing losses, it is equally important that their handicap be identified early to prevent maladjustments and to channel them into an educational program adapted to their needs and directed toward helping them minimize the handicap.[3] The problems centered around hearing impairment in children are not, in any sense, limited to the dysfunction of the hearing mechanism. This is just the cause of the disability. The basic concern is the child's ability to orient himself in the society of the community in which he lives in terms of being able to communicate fully and adequately with others, communication being a much more inclusive concept than hearing and fundamental in all human behavior.

Teacher observation, while helpful, does not always reveal which children have hearing defects. Waldman, in an investigation of the ability of classroom teachers to recognize hearing loss, found that teachers named only 14 out of a group of 63 children with significantly impaired hearing. In addition, teachers listed 46 normally hearing children as defective.[4] Curry, in a similar study, found that teachers referred for hearing tests only 7.4 per cent of the total number of children who might be expected to have a hearing loss.[5] Thus, the need for an objective, standardized test is obvious.

THE SPEECH PHONOGRAPH AUDIOMETER

In about 1926 the speech phonograph audiometer was introduced, and for nearly twenty years was the most popular instrument for screening tests of hearing. This instrument, principally the Western Electric Model 4-C, consisted of a portable phonograph with connections for ten to forty earphones. When the test record was played, the numbers recorded on the disc were transmitted to the receivers, and the numbers became fainter and fainter by three-decibel steps until the threshold for normal hearing was reached. The children listening with the receivers wrote on the test forms as many numbers as they heard. Use of the speech phonograph audiometer has been largely discontinued with the development of more efficient methods of screening.

This test was easy to administer for children above the third grade level, but scoring was tedious and there were many possible sources of error. Repeated studies have demonstrated that this was not an accurate means of detecting hearing loss. For example, a child with reasonably normal hearing in the low frequencies but with a middle and high frequency loss, when listening to the word "two" could record the number correctly on his test form. Because of the nature of his hearing loss, what he actually heard was "oo" without the voiceless consonant "t," and his high frequency hearing loss would go unnoticed. The skill and speed required in recording responses made it unsuitable for children at first and second grade levels.

THE PURE TONE AUDIOMETER

Before the days of electronic audiometers, the problem of testing hearing was relatively simple. The otologist used a tuning fork, watch tick or his whispered voice as the reference standard. What he could hear, he believed his patient should also hear. However, physicians were no more immune to hearing loss than their patients, the intensity of sounds emanating from the tuning fork or watch tick varied greatly, and environmental sounds were not taken into account, so that altogether these early measures were highly inaccurate.

The pure tone audiometer, an electronic instrument for measuring the acuity and range of hearing, provided a major part of the solution to the problem of identifying children with hearing loss. The results of audiometric tests also gave a valid basis for referring children with loss for medical evaluation and possible educational care. The pure tone audiometer is a vacuum tube audio-oscillator equipped to produce tones of fixed frequencies at measurable intensity levels. The frequencies range from approximately 100 cycles per second to 12000 cycles per second at octave or half octave intervals. The tones generated by the audiometer and delivered to the listener by a receiver are of calibrated intensity and measured in decibels, the decibel being defined as the minimum change in intensity which the normal ear can detect in either increasing or decreasing loudness.

The audiometer has two principal controls, the hearing loss dial and the frequency control. At present, standard audiometers use the frequencies 128, 250, 500, 1000, 2000, 3000, 4000, 6000, 8000 and 12000. The hearing loss dial regulates the intensity of each test tone in a range of decibel reference levels from normal hearing to maximum loudness. Readings from this dial are in five-decibel steps.

In addition to these two controls, the off-on switch, the earphone switch, tone interrupter and air conduction-bone conduction switch are also found on the panel. Other dials for regulating masking or speech monitoring may be present on certain models.

Auspices of Screening Program

In urban areas, hearing test services may be a part of the community health program or they may be provided in the schools by the department of education. In rural areas and small communities, routine screening of school age children poses special problems of equipment, personnel and travel. In some states audiometers and audiometric technicians may be

borrowed by the local school district from the state department
of health or education. In several states the problem has been
met by using sound-treated trailers as mobile testing units
which move from community to community.

The decision as to which test should be used in a given school
or community or how the screening program and follow-up
should be carried out can best be made by a professional advisory
committee composed of otologists, audiologists, school medical
staff, educators and representatives of the community health
service. This group should be concerned not only with the type
of screening, but also with a long-range plan of follow-up services. This will bring up for discussion the methods to be used
for retesting children who fail the first test; establishing criteria
for otologic referral; provision of further audiometric study and
otologic diagnostic evaluation; investigating community resources to provide medical care for children from needy
families; and investigating community services for children who
need special educational provision because of irreversible hearing loss.

Testing Personnel

The agency, school or health services designated to assume
responsibility for the hearing screening must provide a suitably
trained staff to administer the tests. The testing is done most
effectively by an audiometrist, one who is equipped by education and experience to give screening and threshold acuity tests.
The audiometrist usually has completed a course sequence in
audiometry or audiology at a recognized college or university,
and in some states is required to have a certificate from the
state department of education. Where the certificate is not required, the American Speech and Hearing Association has established qualifications for persons working in this field.

In schools where the services of a qualified audiometrist are
not available, hearing testing may be done by someone with
less training. Any competent teacher, nurse or even a volunteer
can learn to administer a hearing screening test reasonably well.
A short, intensive in-service training course from a qualified
audiologist or audiometrist is essential, and the less qualified

person will need to work under the supervision of the audiologist. Short courses in audiometry are sometimes offered, as needed, by state departments of health or education or at a nearby college or university. Under no circumstances should an inexperienced individual begin a testing program with no more instruction than is available from an audiometer salesman or a manufacturer's manual.

It is usually not advisable that the time of public health nurses, teachers and speech therapists in the schools be used for conducting routine hearing tests in the schools, as they have responsibilities to carry out more specific to their training. They should, however, be familiar with the screening methods so that they may in turn interpret the program to children and parents. They also have an important role in interpreting test results and in developing effective follow-up procedures.[1]

RECOMMENDED INTERVALS FOR SCHOOL HEARING TESTS

The desirable frequency of hearing tests has not been definitely determined. Practices range from a test for every child each year to tests at two or three year intervals or only on referral by the teacher. There is considerable evidence that most hearing losses in children are acquired rather than congenital, so that a normally hearing child may at any time incur a loss through disease or accident. Wishik and Kramm, in a study of current programs of audiometric testing, suggested that biennial testing of the first through the sixth grade was justified, with junior and senior high grades being tested less often. They found 6.5 per cent of children tested in the first six grades failed the test and suggested that it is unlikely that annual testing would detect a sufficient number of additional cases to warrant a more frequent schedule.[6]

It is important that the screening be done regularly in an established pattern. Some schools test alternate grades each year beginning with grade one. Others test the entire school population every second or third year. In general, it is desirable to test each child biennially in the lower grades and less frequently in the upper grades. Regardless of the intervals for routine screening the plan should be sufficiently flexible to include any child when there is reason to suspect impaired hearing. Each year there should also be added to the regular lists of children to be tested routinely those from other grades who:

are new to the school;

have repeated a grade, or who are doing poorer school work than formerly;

have defective speech, either organic (cleft palate, cerebral palsy) or functional (infantile speech);

showed borderline hearing acuity the previous year;

are subject to colds or ear infections; and those who

have had severe illness or more than the average number of absences.

THE PURPOSE OF PURE TONE HEARING SCREENING

The purpose of the screening test is to provide a rapid, accurate method of determining whether a child has hearing which falls within normal limits or whether hearing loss requiring a more detailed study is present. The results of the screening cannot in themselves be used as a basis for stating that a child has subnormal hearing. Results may indicate that those children screened out require further audiometric study which may show the need for medical referral. A child may fail to respond to the screening because he did not understand the directions, was shy, immature or frightened, or occasionally because the audiometer was defective. Many unfortunate misunderstandings result when parent, teacher or physician are informed that a child had a hearing loss as a result of the screening, when actually his failure to respond to the test was for other reasons.

TESTING CONDITIONS

Hearing tests, to be valid, must be given in a relatively noise-free room. Most newer schools which are equipped with acoustic tiled ceilings meet this requirement. In older, noisy or crowded schools some provision must be made to overcome the environ-

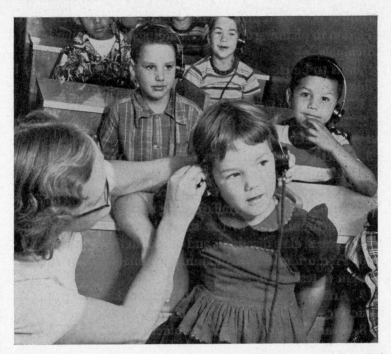

Preparing for the group hearing test. Most children enjoy having their hearing tested, and the experience can be used by the classroom teacher as an opportunity to discuss ears and sound. (Photo courtesy Santa Clara County, California Schools)

mental noise. As a rule, a room on the top floor of the building on a side away from street or playground sounds is most desirable. Rooms adjacent to shops, lavatories, gymnasiums, furnace rooms or music rooms are to be avoided. Occasionally certain uncontrollable noise such as from aircraft or nearby industrial plants makes it desirable to set up the test equipment in another school, nearby church or community hall, and transport the children to the test situation.

PLANNING WITH THE SCHOOL ADMINISTRATION

No successful testing program can be carried out without initial planning with the school administration and clearing all details with principals and teachers of the various schools. Cooperation is assured and interest sustained when there is participation in planning and understanding of the testing by these individuals.

Details to be cleared with the school administration may be as follows:

1. Selection of tentative dates for testing.

2. Announcement of grades to be tested and explanation of test at a teachers' meeting.

3. Selection of a quiet test room. It is well for the audiometric technician to examine the test room in advance and during school hours to make certain it meets the requirements.

4. Reduction of hall traffic during testing.

5. Synchronization of test schedule with school system of bells, recesses, class dismissals and other interference factors.

6. Precautions for maintaining reasonable quiet in rooms adjacent to test room.

7. Arrangement for quiet activities for classes in gym, shop, music, etc., which might disturb testing.

8. Availability of two or more older students or PTA volunteers to assist the audiometric technician.

9. Make certain test dates do not conflict with scheduled school assembly programs, field trips, etc.

10. Suggest that teachers accompany their classes to test room to observe test procedure.

11. Discuss with teachers how hearing test can be utilized as a learning experience related to sound, ears, etc.

12. Discuss method for reporting children screened out as needing further study.

INDIVIDUAL PURE TONE SCREENING

Individual pure tone screening, sometimes called the pure tone sweep check, consists of presenting a series of six to eight test frequencies to the child. These tones will be just barely audible to him in each ear if he has normal hearing. The following procedure, using any standard audiometer, is suggested:

Children may come to the test room in groups of five or six. This saves the technician needless repetition of the test instructions. Children should bring with them a test form, filled out by himself or the teacher in his classroom, with such information as name, age, grade, school and any other desirable information. The student helpers or PTA volunteers may assist in escorting the children to and from the test room, and in seeing that no

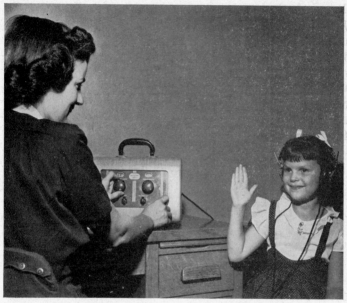

Screening test with the sweep check technique.

time is lost between groups. The child being tested should be seated so that he cannot see the panel of the audiometer. If the audiometer has a single receiver which the child must hold to his ear, sit him at a table or in an armchair. This will give him an opportunity to rest his elbow, thus reducing the possibility of fatigue. For very young children it is advisable for a helper to hold the earphone for the child. Most audiometers have two receivers with a connecting headband making a double head-set. This increases the ease and efficiency in giving the test. In either case, girls may need to push their hair away from under the receiver. The person giving the test should be pleasant and unhurried. Test directions may be as follows:

WE ARE GOING TO PUT ON THE EARPHONES AND LISTEN TO SOME LITTLE SOUNDS. THEY ARE NOT VERY LOUD SO YOU WILL HAVE TO LISTEN CAREFULLY. WHEN YOU HEAR THE SOUND HOLD UP YOUR HAND LIKE THIS (demonstrate). AS SOON AS THE SOUND GOES OFF, PUT YOUR HAND DOWN. YOU MUST SIT QUIETLY WHILE YOU ARE WAITING YOUR TURN. READY NOW, LET'S LISTEN.

Testing Procedure

1. Place the headset on the child and set the earphone switch on the panel of the audiometer to direct the tone to the right ear.

2. See that the tone is off, set the hearing loss dial at the 30 decibel level and the frequency dial at 2000. Throughout the test the hearing loss dial will be set at 15 decibels. The first tone is presented at the 30 decibel level, loud enough to give the child an idea of what the test tone sounds like. The frequency 2000 is used since it is above the level of most environmental noise, thus is easy to hear.

3. Present the tone, using the tone interruptor switch. When the child signals that he hears, interrupt the tone and turn the hearing loss dial to the 15 decibel level. Present the tone again and if the child has normal hearing he should indicate that he hears it.

4. Interrupt the tone, turn the frequency dial to 4000 and present this tone. Proceed in the same manner through the tones 8000, 12000, 1000, 500, 250, 125, thus testing eight frequencies at the 15 decibel level.

5. Test the left ear in the same manner. It may not be necessary to present the first tone at the 30 decibel level. The audiometrist may do so, however, if the child indicates that he does not hear the first tone.

6. If all tones are heard at the 15 decibel level, the child has normal hearing. If a child fails to hear two or more tones for either ear at 15 decibels his hearing does not fall within normal limits and he has been screened out.

7. Under certain conditions of unavoidable environmental

noise the tones 250 and 125 may be omitted since they are most likely to be at the level of the school noise and thus difficult for the children to hear. There is evidence which suggests that if hearing is within normal limits at 500 it is also normal at 125 and 250. The tone 2000 and subsequent higher frequencies are used to begin the test since they are well above the level of most environmental noise and thus easier for the children to hear.

8. The audiometrist must guard against conditioning the child to the rhythm of dialing in this type of test. The audiometrist must also guard against looking at the child in anticipation that he will hear the tone, as each new frequency is presented. The child may learn to respond to the mechanics of the test rather than to the test tones. This can be prevented by varying the time interval in presenting each tone by a few seconds, by not looking directly at the child, and by making certain that the child's signals correspond to the actual presentation and interruption of the tone. It is important to recognize that the reaction time in making responses to the tones may vary from child to child.

9. If the child is immature or retarded it may be well to sweep through the tones at the 25 decibel level before giving the test.

10. Scoring is done as the audiometrist makes two piles of the test sheets, one for those children with normal hearing and one for those who have been screened out as having possible loss. When a child fails the test, no mention of the fact need be made to him, thus avoiding any embarrassment for him before the other children and any possible misunderstanding in the event that he has normal hearing on another audiometric test.

11. Test results should be reported to the school administrator and teachers, notations should be made on the pupil health record cards, and arrangements made for follow-up audiometric study of those children screened out.

12. Children with skin conditions or obvious ear disease should be excused from the test without embarrassing them, and a notation of this should be recorded for the school nurse or teacher on the test form.

GROUP HEARING TESTS

Pulse Tone Group Test

Reger and Newby have reported a group pure tone test consisting of a number of pulses of pure tones. The child taking the test responds by recording in the appropriate space on the test form the number of pulses heard at each frequency level tested. The first tone at each frequency level is presented at 40 decibels. Subsequent pulses of this tone are given at 30, 20, 15 and 5 decibels. Each frequency level is presented in this descending pattern by the audiometrist following a predetermined pattern.[6] Test papers are scored by comparing them with the audiometrist's key. Up to 40 children can be tested at one time. Before the test is given, the output of the phones must be determined experimentally as with the Massachusetts hearing test.

Group pulse tone audiometry has been found effective with college students and adults, but is difficult to administer to children. The audiometrist must make rapid adjustments of the frequency and hearing loss dials and of the interruptor switch.

The Massachusetts Hearing Test

This test accomplishes a pure tone screening for ten to forty children simultaneously, depending on the number of receivers used. It was developed by Dr. Philip W. Johnston, Head of the Child Growth and Development Section of the Massachusetts Department of Health, as an outgrowth of a series of test developments during World War II. Equipment consists of a pure tone audiometer with ten to forty single receivers.

The Massachusetts Hearing Test has been discontinued in many areas in favor of the Johnston Group Pure Tone Test, which was subsequently developed by Johnston. This new test overcomes a number of disadvantages and possible sources of error in the Massachusetts Test. In the former test, calibration of the equipment was subjective, and was done by the audiometrist each time the equipment was set up. In its original form the Massachusetts Test used only three frequencies, 500, 4000, 12000; it is entirely possible for a child to have a significant

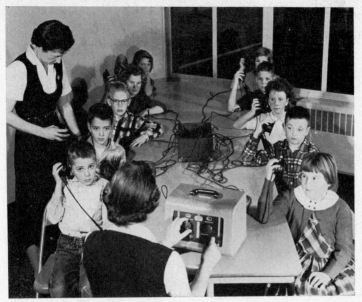

Preparation for the Johnston Test.

hearing loss at the intervals between these tones. The Johnston Test also eliminates scoring of test forms required by the Massachusetts Test.

Johnston Group Pure Tone Test

The objective of this test is to give ten children a group pure tone sweep check with the accuracy approaching that obtained in an individual pure tone sweep check. There are other advantages as follows: (a) no paper or pencils are used by the children; (b) the audiometrist uses basically the same simple procedure used in the individual sweep check; (c) the test is faster and less fatiguing to audiometrist and children; (d) the test is as accurate as the individual sweep check; (e) most portable audiometers can be adapted to a Johnston Test; (f) testing may be done in any room which is quiet and large enough to accommodate table and chairs for ten children; and (g) first-grade children can be tested satisfactorily.

The Johnston Test is not at present produced commercially, but can be made by an electronics laboratory on specifications

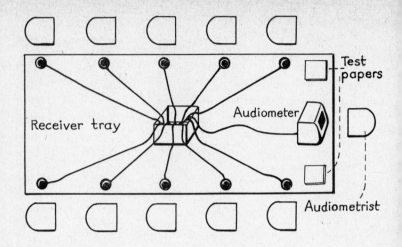

WITH TABLE AND CHAIRS

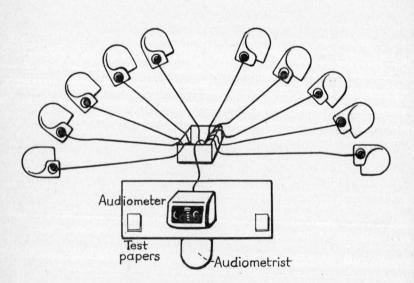

WITH DESK AND TABLET ARM CHAIRS

Arrangement of equipment for the Johnston Test.

from the Massachusetts Department of Health. A standard portable audiometer with bone conduction circuit is modified for use as a multiple audiometer, ten magnetic single receivers, usually Western Electric No. 716A, being added. The instrument thus adapted can no longer be used for bone conduction testing, but the air conduction circuit remains unchanged.[7]

Test Procedure

The planning and test conditions required and setting up equipment are similar to those required for the previous tests. The audiometer is set up on a circular or oblong table with chairs facing the audiometrist. Children come to the test room in groups of ten, and bring with them a test sheet, prepared in their rooms, as in the individual pure tone test. The test sheet may contain such information as name, age, grade, teacher's name, school, etc. When the children are seated around the table, test sheets are collected in the order in which the children are seated. By placing five sheets on either side of the audiometer, each child can be located easily and any notation be made on the proper sheet. The technician may say to the children:

IN A MINUTE WE ARE GOING TO LISTEN TO THE EARPHONES. YOU WILL HEAR A SOUND LIKE THIS. (Turn panel earphone switch to activate one of the individual receivers from the headset of the audiometer, and present one or two high frequency tones at the 90 to 95 decibel level.) EACH TIME YOU HEAR THE TONE HOLD UP YOUR HAND QUICKLY LIKE THIS (demonstrate), AND AS SOON AS THE TONE GOES OFF PUT YOUR HAND DOWN. LET'S PRACTICE. (After a brief practice with one or two tones, turn panel switch to the Johnston Test position.)

PICK UP THE EARPHONE IN YOUR RIGHT HAND AND HOLD IT TO YOUR RIGHT EAR. GIRLS MAY HAVE TO PUSH HAIR BACK OUT OF THE WAY. (Glance quickly around group to see that receivers are held properly to the right ear.) NOW WE ARE READY TO LISTEN, SO SHUT YOUR EYES, KEEP THEM SHUT TIGHT AND WHEN YOU HEAR THE SOUND HOLD UP YOUR HAND.

Turn the frequency dial to 1000 and the hearing loss dial at the 15 decibel level. Proceed with a sweep check of the tones 1000, 2000, 3000, 4000, 6000, 500, and 250. Vary the time interval by two or three seconds by using the tone interruptor. When the right ear has been tested, allow a minute for relaxation, then test the left ear in the same manner. Under certain conditions of unworkable environmental noise the intensity may be increased to 20 decibels, but no more. The increase in intensity should seldom be necessary.

Scoring

All tones must be heard to pass the test. When a child misses a tone, a notation or check should be quickly made on his test sheet. Scoring consists of separating the test sheets for those children screened out as having possible loss from those with normal hearing.

Once or twice during the testing of each group the audiometrist may depress a push button which is wired into the lead to the tray of ten receivers, and concealed from the children. The ten receivers are connected in such a way that when the push button is depressed, two of the receivers are cut off. These receivers are marked with a colored band for quick identification. Removing the tone from the two receivers periodically helps the audiometrist to determine whether the children are giving honest responses.

Other Group Tests

Meyerson has described a group speech audiometric test using simple words containing various English speech sounds. This speech test is administered in recorded form to ten children simultaneously. The children indicate they have heard the word by pointing to the correct picture on the mimeographed test sheet. Meyerson found this method useful in locating children with hearing loss in the speech frequencies.[9]

Individual Versus Group Pure Tone Screening

We recognize that the important first step in case finding is to locate as early as possible the child with actual or potential hearing loss. An efficient hearing test not only identifies children with hearing impairment, it also correctly identifies children whose hearing is normal. The specific method used to achieve this goal will be determined largely by the size of the community and the staff and equipment available.

Group screening, where there are large numbers of children to be tested, is by far the most efficient method. In addition to full utilization of personnel and equipment, it has been established that young children tested in a group are more responsive and less likely to be frightened by the earphones and the test. Individual screening, on the other hand, is most effective for children who are immature, retarded or who have other problems which prevent them from doing their best in a group test.

Follow-up to the Hearing Screening

It is important to record the tests results, normal or otherwise, for each child on his health record card, Wetzil Grid, permanent record, or whatever system is used to keep an anecdotal health history.

In an organized hearing conservation program, the screening is regarded as a means to the end. The quality of the program depends largely on the medical and education resources available for children found to have possible loss, and how these facilities are utilized. Adequate follow-up consists of: (1) further audiometric study to verify and measure the hearing loss as discussed in chapter 4; (2) an otologic diagnostic examination as discussed in chapter 2; (3) special educational care for those children with permanent handicapping losses as discussed in chapters 6, 7 and 8.

When further audiometric study shows a child's hearing to be below normal limits, or when there is an obvious or suspected pathologic disorder of the ear, the parents should be contacted and apprised of the situation. The public health nurse or school nurse is usually available to visit the home to interpret the child's needs and to encourage parents to seek medical advice. The examination may be given on a private basis by a local otologist, in a public health department otologic clinic, at a local children's hospital ear, nose and throat clinic or in some other facility provided by the parents or suggested by the public health nurse. The nurse, when necessary, will encourage and as-

sist parents in planning for recommended treatment. Where
parents are financially unable to provide examination or treatment, the public health nurse usually knows of local resources
to assist the family.

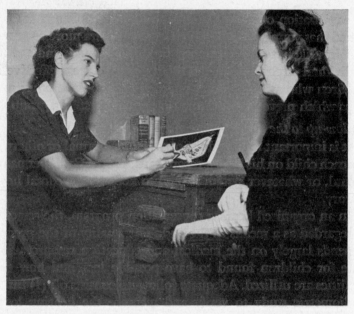

The public health nurse is usually available to interpret the child's needs
to parents, and to encourage parents to seek medical advice.

Children who undergo treatment should then be scheduled
for a recheck hearing test several months after completion of
medical care to redetermine their hearing status. It is encouraging to note that with early discovery and proper medical care,
in most instances, hearing will be normal in the post-treatment
hearing tests. For cases where there is still some loss, the child
should return to the physician for another examination and
possible further treatment.

REFERENCES

1. Services for Children with Impaired Hearing. American Public Health
   Association, Inc., 1790 Broadway, New York 19, N. Y.

2. LANDIS, JAMES E.: A Report on the Hearing Survey in the Public Schools of Pennsylvania. Tr. Am. Acad. Ophth. 56:73–76, 1952.

3. HARDY, WILLIAM G.: Hearing Impairment in Children—A Program for Prevention and Control. A Speech Given at the Audiology Conference University of Washington, December 4, 1950.

4. WARWICK, HAROLD L.: Hearing tests in the public schools of Fort Worth. Volta Review 30:641–643, 1928.

5. CURRY, E. THAYER: The efficiency of teacher referral in a school hearing testing program. J. Speech & Hearing Disorders, 15:211–214, 1950.

6. ROGER, SCOTT N. AND NEWBY, HAYES A.: A group pure tone hearing test. J. Speech & Hearing Disorders. 12:61–66, 1947.

7. WISHIK, SAMUEL M. AND KRAMM, ELIZABETH R.: Audiometric testing of hearing of school children. J. Speech & Hearing Disorders. December, 1953.

8. JOHNSTON, PHILIP W.: An efficient group screening test. J. Speech & Hearing Disorders. 17:8–12, 1952.

9. MEYERSON, LEE: Hearing for Speech in Children: A Verbal Audiometric Test. Unpublished Ph.D. dissertation, Stanford University, 1951.

10. JOHNSTON, PHILIP W.: The Massachusetts hearing test. J. Acoustical Soc. Am. 20:697–703, 1948.

11. NEWBY, HAYES A.: Audiology: Principles and Practice. New York, Appleton-Century-Crofts, 1958.

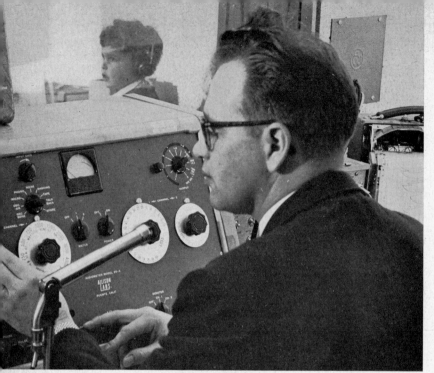

Photo courtesy Washington State Department of Health

4

Clinical Audiometry

MEASURING THE CHILD'S HEARING

AN accurate determination of hearing ability is obviously of the utmost importance when an initial study is being made to determine the reasons why a child's development is not progressing normally and when plans are being made for the education and training of a child known to have some degree of auditory disability. To test hearing with precision is unfortunately not easy, especially with young children and those who have been acoustically handicapped since birth or early infancy.

74

Nevertheless, every possible effort must be made to arrive at an explicit evaluation of how well the child hears, since such clinical information is absolutely basic.

The specialist—medical or educational—will naturally need specialized techniques and information for the hearing examination; the parent or teacher should have a knowledge of these procedures which is sufficiently detailed to enable him to understand the significance of what he is told about the child's hearing. In some situations it is necessary also for the teacher or parent to have enough insight to judge whether or not the examinations which have been conducted are adequate. The present chapter will discuss the methods of estimating hearing loss in children, with particular emphasis on orientation information for therapists, teachers and parents.

HEARING AND THE PERCEPTION OF SPEECH

Before going on to a specific explanation of the various ways in which hearing can be tested and measured it will be helpful to understand some background material which will throw light on the reasons for certain test procedures. Many of the terms which are used also require definition. It should be realized that the primary reason for evaluating a child's hearing is to determine how well he can hear and understand speech. Of course, he needs to be able to hear other kinds of sounds in the environment but if his hearing is adequate for communication he will also be able to hear other environmental sounds satisfactorily. Likewise, when a clinical study is being made of a child who does not seem to hear, an actual sensory loss is not the only possible reason for his behavior. The present discussion will, however, be confined to the role of the sense of hearing itself in the perception of speech.

As pointed out in Chapter 2, normal hearing for speech and other sounds requires that the ear be normally sensitive over a fairly wide range of sound frequencies. As is well known, sound is a form of wave motion; and the *frequency* of a sound is the number of sound waves per second being created by the sound source (measured in cycles per second, cps). In listening to sounds one has a certain experience of "highness" or "lowness" which is called the *pitch* of the sound. The sensation of pitch is directly related to the frequency of the sound vibrations. In terms of a physical scale this relationship is as follows:

Frequency	Pitch
128 cps	C_3
256 cps	C_4
512 cps	C_5
1024 cps	C_6
2048 cps	C_7
4096 cps	C_8
8192 cps	C_9

Sounds vary not only in *pitch,* but also in *loudness.* When one uses the term loudness he is referring to a certain aspect of the sound as a sensation or experience. The loudness of a sound is proportional to the amount of physical energy which reaches the hearing mechanism, or to the *intensity* of the sound. If this general principle is understood, the complexities of the relationship between intensity and loudness can be ignored. Hearing losses are commonly expressed in a unit of intensity, the *decibel* (db), although other units of measurement are sometimes used. Thus, one may be told that a child has a 15 db loss, a 60 db loss, and so on. Actually the decibel is a unit for expressing a ratio between, or difference in, the amount of energy in two sounds, in the same manner, for instance, that a "mile" may be used for measuring linear distance between two places. To continue the illustration, if one says "It is 10 miles to Chicago," he is expressing the distance in relation to some point of departure which could be thought of as "0" miles.

The decibel, as used in the measurement of hearing, then, expresses a "sensory distance" in relation to a fixed point of reference which, for purposes of such measurement, has a value of "0." This point of reference is the average *lower threshold of hearing* (commonly called the "threshold of hearing"), or the point at which a sound (of given frequency) is just perceptible to the normal ear. The intensities needed for sounds of various frequencies to be "just heard" by the normal ear have been determined by testing large numbers of persons and by appropriate statistical analysis of the results. This set of values, called the Beasley Scale, is employed in calibration of the pure tone audiometer. If any other type of audiometer is used, a similar set of values must have been determined previously in order that a child can be "tested," or compared to the "normal." In view of the foregoing explanation it is now understood that a child with a 35 db loss cannot hear the sound in question unless its intensity is 35 db greater than would be necessary for the sound to be just audible to the normal ear. The same idea may be expressed by saying that the child's threshold is *raised* 35 db. Conversely, if the child's hearing is more acute than the average, one might be told that his threshold (or "hearing ability") is –10 db, i.e., the sound is barely audible to him when it contains 10 db less intensity than would be needed for it to become audible to the average ear. In this case the threshold is *lowered*. Losses measured in decibels should never be thought of as percentages of loss, for reasons to be mentioned later.

The ability of a child to hear and understand speech and other sounds depends upon a number of factors. Among them is the capacity of the brain to attach meaning to, or to make use of, whatever sensations reach this level. A disorder of this part of the total process could be discovered only indirectly by audiometric testing. There are, however, certain aspects of speech, considered in the sense of a sound stimulus, which must be related to normal function of the ear as a sensory apparatus in order to get a clear understanding of what actually is revealed by audiometric testing.

From a purely acoustic point of view the speech sounds would be considered *complex* sounds. By this is meant that each of the speech elements is a composite of a number of individual or separate sounds (called partials), in the same way that a musical chord might be thought of as a complex tone made up of several notes. When one listens to a piano chord the ear does not normally distinguish the individual tones which make up the whole. Yet the particular notes the chord contains and their relations to one another as to frequency and intensity gives to it the distinguishing characteristics which might enable the trained musician to identify any given arrangement as a "major," "minor," "diminished 7th" or the like.

As with musical chords, each of the speech sounds has a distinctive arrangement of partial vibrations which enable the listener to distinguish it as a particular sound. It follows, therefore, that a child cannot recognize the speech sounds with optimum efficiency unless his hearing is normal for all of the frequencies of which they are composed. It is well known that in certain common types of auditory defects hearing may be better or worse for some frequencies than for others, and that the particular pattern of loss in any case will have an influence on the speech sounds which can or cannot be heard. The relationship between the frequency response of the ear and the perception of the various speech sounds is somewhat complex, but it can be said in general that for optimum efficiency in hearing speech the threshold must be normal for the range between 100 cps and 8000 cps approximately. After speech has been learned and is well established, an older person may suffer some loss at either end of this range without necessarily experiencing a handicapping disability in understanding speech. For such a person the range between 500 cps and 2000 cps is most important. Any loss in the wider range in a child, however, would impose a much greater hearing difficulty, particularly if the defect occurred before speech was well established. The foregoing considerations are among the reasons why the pure tone audiometer was designed to determine the lower threshold of hearing over a wide range of frequencies.

It is possible to make a very approximate grouping of the speech sounds on the basis of their characteristic frequencies. The so-called "high frequency" sounds are usually listed as *s, z, sh, zh, th* as in *th*ink, *th* as in *th*at, *ch* as in *chair, j* as in *Joe, p, b, t, d, f, v* and *h.* Frequencies above 2000 cps carry a significant amount of the energy in these sounds. Sounds within this group might be recognized by a child who did not hear frequencies above 2000 cps, but this would be much more difficult than for a listener with entirely normal hearing. The remainder of the speech sounds carry a large portion of their energy in frequency bands below 2000 cps, although some of them possess frequencies near this level or above. Despite the complicating factors, one may expect a child with a significant loss at 2000 cps or above to have difficulty in identifying and discriminating among the so-called high frequency sounds and to have a corollary difficulty in developing these sounds in his own speech. A child with a loss limited to high frequencies would, however, be entirely aware of speech and somewhat responsive to it, but would have definitely impaired ability to understand. Again, it should be emphasized that regional hearing losses have a different significance for infants and young children than for older children and adults who are experienced listeners.

Another factor which influences the child's ability to understand speech is the fact that the various speech sounds vary quite widely in their relative strength, as articulated by the average speaker, and hence differ in their audibility. This means, of course, that a child with a mild or moderate hearing loss will have more difficulty with the speech sounds of low phonetic power, even though he gets the sounds of greater phonetic power relatively well. In general, the vowels and diphthongs are most audible, while most of the high frequency sounds are in the group with the least phonetic power. Weakest of all is *th* as in *th*ink, closely followed by *f, p, d, b, th* as in *th*at, *v, k, g, t, s, z* and *zh.* (Fletcher)

Special mention should be made of the way in which the ability to understand speech is affected by the age at which the hearing loss is acquired. If an individual's hearing does not become defective until he has reached adult life the effect on his understanding of speech will be minimal. This is easy to understand if we remember that he will have developed a high degree of language ability, consistent with his intelligence, education and the like. Imperfectly heard words may be understood without difficulty, in the same way that one can recognize a familiar figure at great distance. Not only will minimal auditory cues suffice for word recognition, but also meanings will be inferred from the context in which the word appears. Moreover, visual cues—unconscious lip reading—will aid the failing sense of hearing. There are many ways in which the listener may compensate for his sensory loss, such as sitting nearer the front at church and in meetings or classes, moving closer to the speaker, watching his face more carefully, or turning the head to accommodate a better ear. If the onset of the hearing loss is gradual, as it is typically, the adjustment can be made gradually. Even if the onset of the hearing defect is sudden, the person still has well-established language resources which can be utilized on the basis of cues other than those of an auditory nature. Speech in cases of this sort is likely to deteriorate slowly, or not at all, because of the numerous tactual and kinesthetic cues of which the speaker is unconsciously aware.

The child who has been deaf or hard of hearing from birth onward, or who suffers this condition early in life, is in a much different position. In the first place, he will lack those auditory capacities which are essential to the development of speech. In the same way his capacity for general language development—the acquisition of a vocabulary of auditory symbols which carry meaning—will be lessened to the degree that he is unable to hear. The poverty of language will in turn bear a very important relationship to the child's ability to "think" or conceptualize. He is from the very first, or from an early age, quite out of touch with his environment in one critical respect, and the consequences for his social and emotional adjustment are very significant. Such a child does not recognize speech on the basis of partial cues in the same way as would the adult with an equal degree of acquired hearing loss. All of these factors must be kept in mind when one is attempting to determine what effect a hearing loss will have, not only on speech and language development, but also on total behavior and development.

In addition to the *lower threshold of hearing,* which was discussed earlier, there is a threshold of *feeling* for sound and, at slightly higher intensities than the latter, a threshold of *pain.* When, therefore, a sound reaches a sufficient intensity the sensation of hearing changes to one of feeling, which becomes painful if the stimulus is further increased. The useful hearing lies, then, between the lower thresholds of hearing and of feeling. This spread varies with the frequency of the sound, as seen in figure 1. At 125 cps the threshold of feeling is approximately 95 db above the threshold of hearing, whereas at 1000 cps the

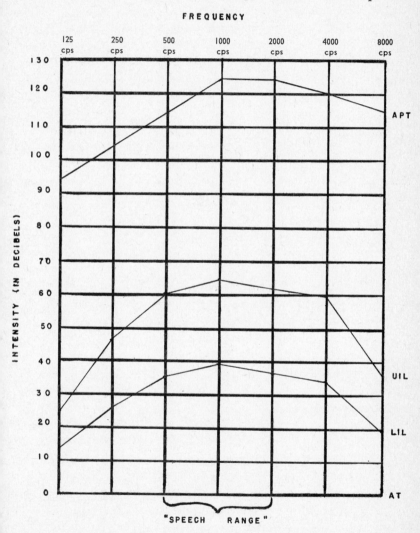

FIG. 1.—Intensity limits of average conversational speech (at 10–20 feet) at frequencies of from 125 to 8000 cps. (APT, approximate pain threshold; UIL, upper intensity limit; LIL, lower intensity limit; AT, average threshold)

distance is about 125 db. The distance decreases somewhat at the upper end of the frequency scale. These facts mean that, in interpreting the audiogram, "deafness" or complete loss of useful hearing will occur at different intensity levels, depending upon the frequency of the sound.

The relation of frequency and intensity factors to the perception of speech is summarized in figure 1. This graph shows the upper and lower intensity limits of average conversational speech at 10 to 20 feet at the various frequency levels. The so-called speech range of 500 cps to 2000 cps is indicated, but one should be reminded that the frequencies above and below this range are important for the child. From the graph it may be seen that at 2000 cps, for instance, average speech sound energy ranges between about 35 and 60 decibels above the normal threshold. The curves slope somewhat downward at either end of the scale. An approximate idea of how much effect a hearing loss may have on the perception of speech for a person with a hearing loss could be gained by visualizing where his threshold of hearing would fall. For example, if there were a straight 30 db loss for all frequencies the lower limit of intensity for average conversational speech would be no more than 10 db above this individual's actual threshold at any point. The upper intensity limit of average conversational speech would be only about 20 db above threshold in the speech range. One would need to consider also the fact that the amount of speech sound energy available to this person would be decreased further by the inevitable presence of masking sounds in the environment.

A final word should be said about the conditions under which the hearing test is made. One of the commonest sources of error is the degree to which test results are falsified by poor test techniques. With children it is obvious that most tests require an understanding of what the examiner wants and a willingness to cooperate. The skilled examiner naturally takes these factors into account in interpreting the test results. If a given test, such as the pure tone audiometer, is judged too complex for the child, the examiner will as a matter of course employ some other technique—perhaps speech audiometry. Although these comments seem obvious, experience shows that in actual practice conclusions are often drawn about a child's ability to hear on the basis of test results which are unreliable for the reasons mentioned. Another evident fact is that great patience is required if one is to test children successfully, and an accurate hearing test sometimes becomes quite time-consuming. Several sessions often are required. Tests given hastily may be quite unreliable. Many times several test sessions on different days will be necessary before a truly accurate audiogram is made. Of great importance also for reliable testing is the amount of noise in the test room. A "sound-proof" or "quiet" room is absolutely essential and such conditions cannot ordinarily be provided without special acoustic treatment to shut out incidental noise in the environment. Even what may seem like a quiet room to the ordinary observer can easily be noisy enough to make a 25 db error in test results. Test conditions in the typical school classroom are notoriously poor. All of these factors must be taken into account in assessing the reliability of any hearing test.

THE MEDICAL EXAMINATION

No hearing evaluation is complete without a careful and thorough otologic examination. This is usually the starting point for the comprehensive study needed for the child who is suspected of having a hearing problem. The purpose of a medical examination is to discover whether or not there is any pathologic abnormality of the hearing mechanism which could lead to an auditory defect, and to evaluate the child's medical history to disclose any past conditions which might have affected hearing. The outstanding diseases of the ear which the otologist looks for have been discussed in Chapter 2. The presence of any of the conditions mentioned there will naturally create the presumption that a hearing loss exists. If the child's behavior and general developmental progress are consistent with this tentative conclusion it usually is best to assume that the child is either hard of hearing or deaf—as circumstances warrant—and to plan his training and management on this basis even though a completely reliable hearing test cannot be carried out. Occasionally the tentative diagnosis proves wrong, or must at least be modified, but in problems of this kind one should rarely hold up training until a completely final diagnosis is made. It goes without saying, of course, that every possible medical resource for the treatment of any hearing loss should be utilized.

There are certain limitations to the information which can be derived from even the most careful and comprehensive medical study. Among the most important of these is the fact that negative medical findings do not necessarily prove that the child has normal hearing. It is quite possible that even a careful otologic examination, except for a hearing test, may prove entirely negative. Nevertheless, a hearing loss may be present. Negative findings so far as demonstrable abnormalities of the hearing mechanism are concerned may mean only that the hearing loss is of a type which cannot be found by any method except that of specialized hearing tests. This point seems clear enough, yet parents are particularly prone to conclude that a child's hearing is normal when they are told that no disease of the ear has been discovered. This often occurs among more poorly informed parents and teachers after a physician, usually in the course of a routine medical check-up, has "looked into the child's ears." Such an examination can, of course, yield information only about the external ear canal and the appearance of the tympanic membranes (eardrums). This does not constitute an adequate otologic examination.

Practice varies among physicians with respect to the administration of extensive hearing tests. Some prefer to confine themselves to certain routine tests which can be carried out in the office without undue expenditure of time, and to refer the child to an audiologic clinic or center for the more detailed hearing tests which are necessary with some of the children who are difficult to test. Other otologists are prepared to conduct comprehensive examinations of hearing function in children of all ages and will do so in their own offices. Stress should be laid on the point that the measurement of hearing is a matter in which the physician and the educational specialist have a joint interest, but with somewhat different foci of emphasis.

The otologist is primarily concerned with discovery of any detectable loss, after which he goes on to the specialized tests which will enable him to form a judgment as to the kind of disorder which is responsible. Such examinations enable him to differentiate between disease of the auditory nerve and inadequate functioning of other parts of the hearing mechanism. They may provide clues as to the particular disorder present. The teacher, however, is more directly concerned with the child's over-all hearing efficiency. The characteristics of the hearing loss govern the way in which the child can be taught to compensate for his lack of hearing or to make better use of any residual hearing he may possess. Often the hearing measurement which is adequate for medical purposes is not sufficient for planning educational therapy.

TUNING FORK TESTS

One of the standard procedures used by the otologist involves certain observations of hearing made by use of tuning forks. Such tests are primarily *qualitative*, that is, they are useful in determining the type of hearing loss which is present. To some extent, and under some conditions, the tuning fork may be used to find out how well the patient hears, but such *quantitative* measurements made in this way are much less satisfactory with children than are other methods to be discussed in later paragraphs. Nevertheless, the parent and teacher should have a general understanding of the commonest tuning fork tests which the otologist may use.

Most otologists make routine use of the Rinne test, which is useful in differentiating defects of the auditory nerve from those of the conducting mechanism (outer and middle ears). It is administered as follows: after the tuning fork is set into vibration its shank is placed firmly immediately behind and toward the upper part of the external ear (on the mastoid portion of the temporal bone). The patient signals as soon as the sound is no longer heard by bone conduction and the prongs of the fork are then immediately placed near the external ear canal. The Rinne is said to be positive if, under these conditions, the sound is heard once more by air conduction. If hearing is normal the sound is heard at least twice as long by air conduction as by bone conduction. The Rinne is positive if the middle ear is functioning normally, but this is not a quantitative test of acuity. On the other hand, the Rinne is negative if the sound is heard better by bone conduction than by air conduction. This may be tested by holding the vibrating fork near the external auditory canal until the sound is no longer heard. The shank of the fork is then placed against the mastoid portion of the temporal bone. If the sound reappears, this demonstrates that bone conduction hearing is relatively better than air conduction hearing; hence, a negative Rinne points to a conductive type of lesion. If the sound is heard longer by air conduction than by bone conduction, but not *twice* as long, an inner ear and conductive loss is inferred. There are many complicating factors in interpreting Rinne findings, but these need not be discussed.

Another observation of the bone conduction hearing of a patient may be made rapidly by use of the Schwabach test. This is administered by placing the shank of a vibrating tuning fork on the bone behind the ear as described for the Rinne test. The fork is held in this position until the bone-conducted sound is no longer heard. The fork is then transferred to a corresponding point on a person with "normal" hearing (usually the examiner). In this way a judgment can be made as to whether the bone conduction hearing of the patient is decreased, normal or increased as compared to that of a normal-hearing individual. If the sound is heard by the normal person after it is no longer sensed by the patient the latter's bone conduction hearing is obviously decreased. There are, of course, many limitations to the usefulness of the Schwabach test.

A third tuning fork test in common use is the Weber test, which is employed for observation of certain variables where unilateral hearing loss is present or suspected. To administer the Weber test, the shank of a vibrating tuning fork is placed on top of the skull at the midline (vertex of the head). When this is done the resulting sound may be heard equally well in each ear or it may be heard relatively better (lateralized) in either the right or left ears. Such lateralization may vary in the degree of certainty with which the patient locates the sound in one of the two ears. In general, a patient with a unilateral conductive hearing loss will localize the sound as being in the diseased ear. If, on the other hand, one ear is affected by a nerve loss (or affected to a relatively greater extent than the other ear) the sound will appear to be localized in the "good" ear. As with other tuning fork tests, there are many special considerations which affect interpretation of the results, and such measurements are significant only in the hands of a skilled and experienced examiner.

There are other examinations which sometimes are performed with tuning forks, but these need not be described in detail in the present discussion. Occasionally, tuning forks are used for at least rough approximations of auditory acuity. Such measurements may be carried out by having the patient signal when he no longer hears the vibrating fork, after which the examiner notes whether or not he himself can hear the sound. Being familiar with the characteristics of his own hearing, the examiner can then make a comparison between himself and the patient, and thus approximate the latter's threshold. This is essentially an "air conduction Schwabach." The number of seconds a vibrating fork can be heard may also be used as a measure of auditory acuity. Tuning forks of different frequencies may be used to determine the acuity of hearing at various pitch levels and to chart roughly the upper and lower frequency limits to which the subject can respond.

It is clear from the foregoing discussion that the various tuning fork tests are primarily diagnostic procedures employed by the otologist as aids in determining the type of hearing loss which may be present. Measurements made in this way do not, however, constitute a "hearing test" in the ordinary sense of the term, and an adequate evaluation of the child's hearing for both medical and educational purposes demands other types of testing to be discussed later. It is obvious also that the validity

and reliability of the tuning fork tests depend upon the extent
to which the child understands what he is being asked to do
and on how well he cooperates. In many circumstances these
tests are of no value with children and, in any event, the parent
and teacher should understand that the child who has had no
other testing has not been diagnosed adequately so far as his
hearing efficiency is concerned. Some otologists have come to
use tuning fork tests very infrequently because they feel the
same information can be brought out more accurately by use
of the audiometer, but the speed and convenience with which
the examination can be made with tuning forks, particularly
with older patients, make these procedures very valuable for
the otologist.

THE PURE TONE AUDIOMETER

The commonest technique in current use for administering
hearing tests for both medical and educational purposes is
audiometry with the pure tone audiometer. In recent years certain other types of audiometry have been developed, but the
pure tone audiometer remains the standard instrument upon
which the diagnostician depends. The importance of audiometry of this type warrants a fairly extensive discussion for the
orientation of parents and teachers.

There are several makes of pure tone audiometers, with differing details of design and operation, but all employ the same
fundamental principles. Basically, the pure tone audiometer
is an instrument which by electronic means produces tones
which can be accurately varied in both frequency and intensity.
This makes it possible for the operator to present to the patient
tones of different pitches, and to increase and decrease the loudness of these tones until he determines the point at which the
sound is "just barely heard." This is the patient's lower threshold of hearing, or in ordinary terms his "hearing ability." The
audiogram is a graph of the threshold of hearing for each ear
at the seven frequencies which are ordinarily included in the
routine test. These are 125, 250, 500, 1000, 2000, 4000 and
8000 cps, although other frequencies may be included. A more

complete discussion of the audiogram will be presented later.

Two kinds of threshold measurements can be made with the pure tone audiometer: *air conduction* and *bone conduction*. Air conduction hearing occurs when the sound enters the ex-

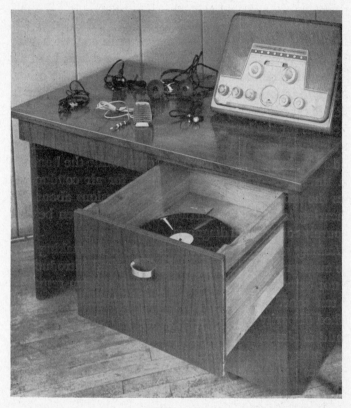

Custom built desk model clinical audiometer with accessories: (left to right) bone conduction receiver, monitor phone, microphone, binaural receivers and patient signal. The turntable attachment is for speech audiometry. (Photo courtesy Corvek Medical Equipment Company, Portland, Oregon)

ternal auditory canal, passes along the sound conducting system of the middle ear and is transmitted to the inner ear with consequent stimulation of the auditory nerve, as explained in Chapter 2. In bone conduction hearing the vibrations pass through the bone containing the ear cavities (temporal bone) to the inner ear fluid, whose movements then result in stimulation of the nerve.

To test air conduction hearing a receiver is placed on the child's ear, after the manner of a radio operator's headset, and the sound is presented in the external ear canal. Some audiometers are equipped with receivers for each ear, with provision for switching from one to the other, while others have a single receiver which must be shifted from one ear to the other. The bone conduction receiver contains a vibrating plate or button which is placed snugly on a selected point on the bone behind the ear, as for the bone conduction tuning fork test. In general, the air conduction threshold gives an over-all measure of the child's hearing efficiency for pure tones, while the bone conduction threshold—when related to that for air conduction—enables the otologist to form certain conclusions about the type of hearing loss. Air conduction testing will often be sufficient for purely educational diagnosis.

Masking sounds are sometimes needed in making the pure tone audiogram. A masking noise is a sound introduced in the ear not being tested in order to prevent it from responding to the test tone. Such masking is quite necessary when there is marked disparity in the acuity of the two ears. If, for example, a child is almost normal in one ear but very hard of hearing in the other ear a tone presented to the poorer ear may, before it reaches the threshold, be loud enough to arouse a response in the better ear. The child will not be aware that this is happening and will report that he hears the sound, presumably in the ear being tested. In the same way vibrations imparted to one temporal bone may pass across the skull to the opposite inner ear above certain intensity levels and lead to spurious test results unless the ear not being tested is "knocked out" by masking.

After the child has been introduced to the audiometer and appropriate explanations and instructions given, the ear phones are adjusted and the actual testing is begun. The general intructions to the child are that he is to signal as soon as the sound is heard, and again when the tone "goes away" or is no longer audible. It is of the utmost importance that the child understand the response he is to make, and herein lies one of the principal difficulties in carrying out pure tone audiometry with some children. The signal itself is a matter of some practical importance. Many audiometers are provided with a switch containing a button, which may be held in the hand, and a signal light which goes on when the button is pressed. Conventionally, the child is asked to turn the light on when the sound is heard and to turn it off when the sound is no longer audible. Such a method of signalling often proves unsatisfactory, and it is usually more convenient to ask the child to hold his hand up while the sound is heard and to put his hand down when the sound is not heard. This type of signal is much more likely to be given reliably. It may even become necessary to ask the child, each time a tone is presented, "Do you hear this?"

There are several ways in which the actual threshold may be determined. In general, of course, the lower threshold of hearing is the point of minimum intensity at which the sound is just perceptible to the child. This figure, it will be remembered, is usually given in terms of the number of decibels above or below the average threshold. A conventional method is to give the child a tone which is thought to be well above his threshold, then to reduce the tone by 5 db steps until it is no longer heard. The lowest intensity level at which the sound can be heard (a value which is read from the hearing loss dial of the audiometer) is the threshold. Most audiometers have a tone interrupter in the form of a switch which cuts off the signal entirely. The tone interrupter also enables the operator to tell whether or not the child is actually responding to the sound. When the sound is switched off the child should, of course, signal at once that he does not hear. In this way the test sound can be presented at each successive intensity level in such a way that there is an interval of silence between test stimuli. This procedure probably elicits the most reliable response from the child, although some examiners prefer to reduce the intensity of the tone without interrupting it completely. After a few trials the operator usually succeeds in locating the threshold tentatively, and the testing can begin at some convenient level, perhaps 15 or 20 db above what seems to be the child's approximate hearing level. The same general procedures may be used in approaching the threshold from below, i.e., the operator starts testing with tones too weak for the child to hear and increases the intensity, usually by 5 db steps, until the sound is heard.

Sometimes it will be desirable to chart the threshold in both ways. Once the threshold is located, the audiogram blank is marked with the appropriate symbol. A red circle is used to record for the right ear, a blue X for the left ear. The marks are placed at the appropriate intersection of the frequency and intensity lines on the audiogram blank. Other symbols are used for bone conduction threshold tabulations. The marks may be connected by lines to form a graph or profile of the threshold at the frequencies tested, if one finds this easier to read in inspecting the audiogram. The order in which the frequencies are presented is possibly not a matter of great importance, but the usual recommendation is to start with 1000 cps, then work downward to the lowest frequency, usually 125 cps, and conclude with the frequencies above 1000 cps. All pure tone audiometers have a plainly marked control for selecting the frequency.

The child's true threshold at any given frequency is considered to be the minimum intensity level at which he consistently reports that he "just hears" the sound. When stimuli of decreasing intensity are used, this is the level at which he gives the last affirmative signal; if stimuli of increasing intensity are being presented, the threshold is the point at which he gives the first affirmative signal. The number of trials necessary to elicit a reliable response will depend to a large extent on the child—his attention span, the degree of motivation, how well he understands what is wanted, and the like. Under favorable circumstances no more than perhaps three or four trials will be necessary at each frequency; in other cases the utmost patience and repeated trials will be necessary. It is wise to recheck frequencies which yield doubtful findings. The experienced audiometrist will, by careful observation of the child's behavior, be able to form a good judgment as to the reliability of the child's responses. Where his responses are inconsistent, nothing better than an approximate threshold can be determined. Under good test conditions, and with a skilled examiner, threshold measurements may be considered accurate within a plus or minus 5 db range.

In actual practice, however, there are many limitations to the results routinely obtained by pure tone audiometer tests, particularly with children. A first question which must be raised in this connection is the age at which pure tone audiometry is suitable for children's testing. There obviously can be no universally reliable statement on this point. The critical factors are whether or not the child's understanding is sufficiently good for him to comprehend clearly the nature of the test, the kind of response he is supposed to make and whether or not his interest and motivation can be sustained for a long enough period. It is not unusual to find children four years of age or younger who can be examined quite satisfactorily with the pure tone audiometer if the examiner is patient and accustomed to working with children; on the other hand, a much older child with different behavior characteristics may not be suitable for testing of this type.

There are a number of superficial errors in technique which may completely falsify the audiogram. Such mistakes are inexcusable, yet they occur often. One of the commonest is "cueing" the child. For instance, if the youngster is placed in a position where he can watch the operator adjust the controls of the instrument, he is quite likely to signal that he hears at what could be appropriate times. Further, the audiometrist may look expectantly at the child after the intensity of the tone has been adjusted, and this quite naturally leads to a response. Pure tone tests with children cannot be hurried; sufficient time must be allowed at each presentation of the test stimulus for the child to make a judgment, but this is not always done. Examiners sometimes fall into a kind of "rhythm" in the series of test tones and the child may likewise signal at intervals in such a manner as to make it appear that he is responding to the test signal when actually he is not. These and other similar defects in technique must be scrupulously avoided if the audiogram is to be meaningful.

The possibility of intermittent hearing losses caused by such factors as upper respiratory tract infection must also be considered. A word should be said about maintenance of the audiometer itself. The modern instrument is quite rugged, yet like any other electronic device it can be broken or go out of adjustment. One of the most vulnerable parts of the whole system is the earphone, which is sometimes subjected to a great deal of abuse. When an instrument is *calibrated* at the factory before delivery the intensity of the output is carefully adjusted to conform to the Beasley scale, mentioned earlier. If electric or mechanical failure occurs the instrument may drift off scale, with the consequence that it becomes an inaccurate measuring device. Audiometers may also become noisy in such a way as to interfere with the test tone. The audiometrist maintains a reasonably good check on calibration if he becomes thoroughly acquainted with his own hearing, which is then used as a basis for determining periodically the characteristics of any given audiometer. In most situations recalibration of the audiometer must be done by the manufacturer either at the factory or at an established service branch.

Interpreting the Audiogram

Interpreting an audiogram is a task for a medical specialist or for a thoroughly trained audiologist with the necessary special information at his command. Nevertheless, the parent or teacher should acquire the basic knowledge which is needed for understanding audiologic reports. A detailed and comprehensive discussion of these matters cannot be given here, but the following paragraphs should be helpful in understanding in at least a general way what various types of audiograms mean in terms of the child's ability to use hearing for purposes of communication.

The medical diagnostician is naturally interested in the

child's over-all hearing efficiency, but he also is directly concerned with a discovery of the cause of the hearing loss in order that all possible treatment can be given to conserve or improve the child's auditory acuity. The pure tone audiogram is an important aid in such diagnosis, inasmuch as certain patterns of loss revealed in this way are characteristic of specific pathologic of the hearing mechanism. The differential diagnosis of conductive and nerve losses has been mentioned several times. In Audiogram A * is the typical case of a child with nerve im-

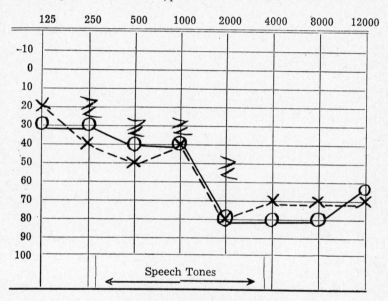

AUDIOGRAM A: Nerve Loss

pairment of unknown origin. Note that the thresholds for bone and air conduction do not differ to any significant extent. The hearing is not significantly improved, as compared to air conduction, when the stimulus is carried to the nerve endings by bone conduction; the auditory nerve is therefore not functioning normally and a nerve involvement must be assumed.

* In this and in the succeeding audiograms the following symbols are used. Air Conduction: right ear = O, left ear = X; Bone Conduction: right ear = >, left ear = <.

In Audiogram B, on the other hand, the bone conduction threshold for both ears is approximately normal, yet the air conduction threshold is raised by a considerable amount. This discrepancy indicates a conductive defect, since the child's hearing is nearly normal when the outer and middle ears are by-passed through the use of a bone conduction receiver.

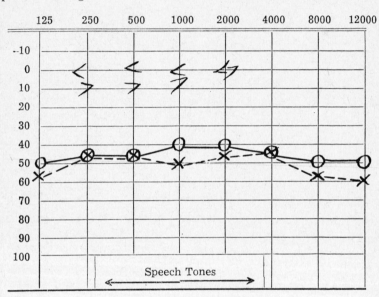

AUDIOGRAM B: Conductive Loss

There are numerous other audiometric findings which will be meaningful to the otologist in terms of specific ear diseases. Our primary interest, however, lies in the different patterns of air conduction loss, since these reflect upon the child's ability to hear and understand speech and other environmental noises. Audiogram C is that of a child with what might be termed a mild hearing loss (probably conductive). The threshold for the right ear is somewhat better than for the left ear, but not significantly so. In general, the loss ranges from 10 to 25 db and is about the same for all frequencies; the audiogram would be called essentially "flat." At the so-called speech frequencies (500,

1000 and 2000 cps) the average loss is between 15 and 20 db. This child, then, will hear conversational speech relatively well under favorable conditions, but will experience difficulty in the presence of any masking noise. And it must be remembered that most of his listening, at school and elsewhere, will be done in

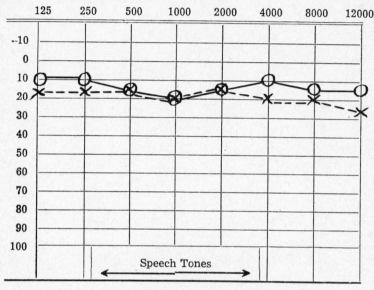

AUDIOGRAM C: Mild Hearing Loss

the presence of a considerable amount of extraneous environmental sound. Child "C" will really never hear with ease and will probably depend unconsciously on speech reading to supplement his sense of hearing. If the hearing loss was present at birth or had an early onset, this youngster may well have been somewhat slow in learning to talk, and may also have exhibited more than the usual number of sound substitutions and other articulatory errors because of his reduced ability to discriminate among the speech sounds. His behavior may have been affected in other ways. Nevertheless, the hearing loss is not really a serious one and conceivably could go undiscovered if he attended a school where routine audiometric examinations were not given, or if some perceptive adult did not suspect the problem. Although not serious, the loss is important and demands careful attention by both medical and educational specialists.

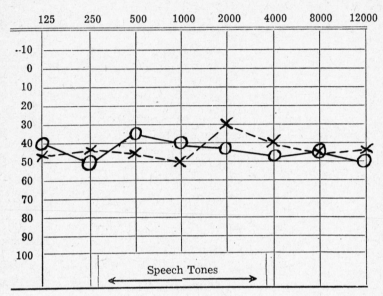

AUDIOGRAM D: Hearing Loss of Moderate Severity

Audiogram D is the hearing test result of a child with a moderately severe loss which will impose a significant handicap. As with child "A," there is an essentially "flat" audiogram, and both right and left ears are involved to an approximately equal degree. The extent of the rise in threshold varies from 30 to 50 db and would average about 40 db for either ear for all seven frequencies. At the speech frequencies the average loss is about 40 db. This child, therefore, will hear speech with great difficulty under favorable conditions. Even where there is no interfering noise and when the child is listening most attentively he will miss a great deal of what is said. In any ordinary environmental situation the child will be very definitely out of touch with the speaker. Child "D" will depend to a great extent upon visual cues in the perception of speech. Loud sounds around him—automobile horns and the like—will be heard, but he will miss many sounds of lesser intensity. Assuming the loss to have been present very early in the child's life, there is almost certain to be a history of marked delay in beginning to talk, and subsequent language development will probably have been slow. The child's articulation problem is likely to be severe.

It is also quite probable that his behavior will be typical for this degree of loss. He almost certainly will not be doing well in school and may even have been mistaken for a mentally defective child, no matter what his actual intelligence may be. He will be understandably inattentive and, depending on the manner in which he has been handled, there may be severe emotional stresses which are reflected in behavior problems. His social and emotional growth can scarcely have been normal. If the loss does not yield to medical treatment, the most careful and comprehensive educational measures will be needed to see this child through his difficulties, probably including amplification in the form of a hearing aid. If the child is otherwise normal, however, he probably can compensate very successfully for a loss of this degree if he gets the needed help. Even if medical treatment improves the threshold significantly, this youngster will for a time need educational therapy to enable him to make up for what he missed during the time the hearing loss was present.

Audiogram E shows the hearing profile of a profoundly hard of hearing child. The problems here have much in common with those of the truly *deaf* child who has no hearing which is useful for purposes of communication. The audiogram would have been equally typical if it showed no response at all at some frequencies—perhaps those at 4000 and 8000 cps. Note that the loss in each ear is no less than 60 db at any frequency and that at 1000 cps the threshold is 85 db. The average loss in the three speech frequencies is nearly 80 db. Note also that throughout the range of frequencies tested the lower threshold of hearing is very close to the threshold of feeling, or the upper limit of hearing.

For all ordinary purposes child "E" is getting virtually no

usable sound. He will sense very loud noises, but will not hear a large proportion of ordinary environmental sounds, such as a telephone ringing in another part of the house, quiet voices and the like. The child may respond if spoken to in a loud tone, but speech will be virtually meaningless because of the severity of the loss unless the loudness level is extraordinarily high. Developmentally there will have been profound delay in the acquisition of "speech," and he may indeed be, for all practical purposes, entirely without speech or have only a rudimentary kind of oral language with a great deal of vocalization but few recognizable words.

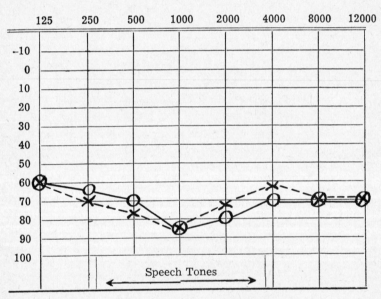

AUDIOGRAM E: Severe Hearing Loss

We would expect this child to fit into a typical pattern. If the loss was present at birth there is a good chance that it will have remained undiscovered until the child passed the age when he should have shown evidences of developing speech. The mother may or may not have noted that the baby failed to awaken in the presence of sounds or respond to loud noises by crying, turning his head, or in some other way. When the suspicion that something was wrong did arise, the physician and other specialists who examined the child may have found it very difficult to reach an exact diagnosis, and the task of excluding intellectual defect or brain damage may have been particularly hard. As time passed, during the preschool years, the child may have grown into a "problem," exhibiting behavior traits of the rejected, and other evidences of emotional disturbance, particularly if the nature of his difficulty has not been understood; or he may, under wise guidance, have developed a better pattern of social adjustment. In any case, he will be operating under the influence of a sensory loss which deprives him of a most important contact with the world. A child of this sort will demand extensive special training and merits the most careful study by the necessary medical and educational consultants. Their recommendations must be followed closely, and the general guidance program should be instituted at the earliest possible age. Early diagnosis is of the utmost importance.

Audiogram F is that of a child with a marked high frequency hearing loss. The threshold at the lower frequencies is nearly normal, but the curve slopes downward in a characteristic way. At 2000 cps. the loss has reached 45 and 40 db in the right and left ears respectively, and the threshold drops another 20 to 30 db at the two upper frequencies. In some cases the audiogram may be still flatter and closer to the normal at the lower frequencies, but drop off even more sharply at 4000 and 8000 cps. Many times the curve rises at 8000 cps. Usually high frequency losses in children are caused by nerve damage.

The speech reception of child "F" will contain certain peculiarities. This youngster will be entirely aware of speech, since his hearing in the lower frequencies is relatively well preserved. Moreover, his understanding will be fairly good in some respects, since his threshold is not severely raised for the frequencies which contain a good deal of the energy of the vowels, diphthongs, certain of the sounds such as *l, m, r* and others which are sometimes thought of as consonants. Even at 2000 cps, which is an important frequency region for the high frequency consonants, acuity is down only 45 db. Nevertheless, speech will

lose a considerable amount of intelligibility for him because
of the drop in acuity at 2000 cps and in the higher frequencies.
Here is an instance in which the child's previous learning will

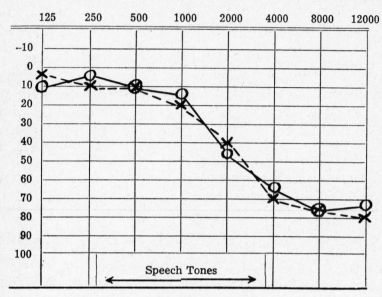

AUDIOGRAM F: High Frequency Hearing Loss

play a very important role. An adult with a loss of this degree
and type which had a relatively late onset might experience
very little difficulty in understanding people, particularly if he
can watch them closely, as he unconsciously will. The younger
child would have somewhat more trouble in discrimination,
however, and if the loss was present before speech became well
established the effect on understanding would be most marked.
In the latter case the articulatory problem of the youngster
would likely be severe, perhaps with particular difficulty on the
high frequency consonants. Very young children with high frequency losses often present puzzling diagnostic problems, since
they seem to hear but do not behave with understanding. Such a
pattern may sometimes be mistaken for intellectual defect or
it may lead to a diagnosis of "children's aphasia" on the assump-

tion that some of the higher language processes are disturbed by brain damage.

In these sample audiograms the thresholds in right and left ears are shown as being much the same, but children often have a loss in one ear with comparatively good acuity on the other side. This raises the question as to how well the child actually hears. For some purposes it is substantially correct to say that hearing efficiency is determined by the threshold in the better ear, and that one defective ear does not impose any great disability on the listener. This should not be assumed as a true statement concerning children, however, since there is abundant clinical evidence that binaural hearing is more efficient than hearing with a single ear. Thus, even if the threshold is normal or nearly so in the right ear, any significant loss in the left ear will make it more difficult for the child to hear with maximum efficiency. His over-all threshold will, however, be fairly close to the threshold for the better ear.

SPEECH AUDIOMETRY

Widespread use has been made in recent years of another method of testing called speech audiometry. This technique is based on the simple principle of using speech itself as the testing stimulus. The result is a direct measurement of the child's hearing efficiency for speech. In some respects speech audiometry is much more satisfactory than pure tone audiometry for use with children, not only because it gives a direct measure of speech perception, but also because the kind of response the child makes—such as identifying pictures whose names he hears—is more interesting to him and easier to understand. A complete hearing evaluation may, of course, include both pure tone and speech audiometry, as well as other types of observation.

The instrumentation necessary for speech audiometry is quite simple in principle, although fairly elaborate equipment and facilities are needed for a really efficient and accurate system. Two sound-treated rooms are needed. One is the test room in which the child is placed (usually accompanied by an assistant to the audiometrist); the second room contains the audiometric equipment with which the operator is working. Conventionally a window is placed at an appropriate point to permit the audiometrist to watch the child during the testing. A "talk-back" system is installed so the audiometrist may hear what is said in the test room. Several of the pure tone audiometers are equipped with "speech circuits" and microphone, and some speech audiometry can be done in this way, but such a provision is far from ideal for good speech testing.

The speech audiometer is basically a high quality public address system with the necessary amplifiers and other components. It is important that the frequency response of the system be essentially flat, i.e., that it reproduce speech with a high degree of fidelity and not introduce the distortion which would result if some of the frequencies were transmitted better than others. The speech audiometer should also have adequate power, or gain, so that sounds can be delivered at intensities of perhaps 100 db or more above the average threshold. Suitable controls are provided so that the intensity of the test sounds can be accurately controlled, usually in 1 db steps. Provision for masking is desirable.

The child may listen to the sounds under several conditions. Earphones may be used, which will permit the examiner to test each ear separately and also to determine how well the child hears binaurally. The sounds may also be presented through a loud speaker in what is called *free field* testing. While this gives only an over-all measure of hearing efficiency and does not enable the audiometrist to measure hearing in each ear individually, it nevertheless is very useful with children who may be afraid of the earphones which must be worn on the head. Free field testing also has many special uses, such as in evaluating the amount of help a child may be getting from a hearing aid. Unlike the pure tone audiometer, there is no set of threshold intensities which can be used in all speech audiometer systems. Instead, each facility has to be individually calibrated, but this can be done with relative ease by using an adequate sized group of subjects with normal hearing. The test material may be presented either by live voice or from tape or phonographic recordings. In live voice testing the operator speaks into a microphone. With adequate practice the audiometrist learns to keep variations in the intensity of his speech within allowable limits, and he usually has a monitoring meter which makes it possible for him to keep a visual check on this factor. The phonographic or tape recordings are, of course, fed directly into the amplifying system.

A wide variety of material is used for testing with the speech audiometer. With somewhat older children and adults extensive use is made of the so-called Harvard Word Lists, which have been standardized for articulation tests. Most speech audiometer testing is carried out in a simpler way with very young children. A number of pictures are placed before the child and he is asked to point to the appropriate picture when it is named. The examiner then calls the names of the pictures at varying levels of intensity until the threshold is determined. This gives a direct measure, usually expressed in decibel units, of the child's ability to hear speech. The level at which the child responds correctly 50 per cent of the time is called the *speech reception threshold*. This is somewhat above the *threshold of detectability*, which is the point at which the speech is heard but not necessarily understood.

The foregoing description of speech audiometry does not give an adequate idea of the various technical aspects of selection of test material and other details which are involved. Properly employed, however, the thresholds derived from speech audiometry may be considered fully as reliable as are the responses in pure tone audiometry, and the measurements are no less precise. A complete diagnostic examination will ideally include both pure tone and speech testing.

One of the particular values of speech audiometry with children is the fact that they generally find the situation less threatening, so that the timid child responds better. Furthermore, the activity of looking at pictures is more familiar and pleasurable, hence interest and effort are more easily sustained. The nature of the task is less complex, hence the responses made by certain types of children may be much more reliable than in pure tone audiometry. The age level at which testing can be successfully carried out is generally much lower for speech audiometry, especially for children who are difficult to test. Children who cannot be tested in other ways because of language deficiencies may sometimes be reached through the speech audiometer by first spending whatever time is necessary to teach them the names of pictured objects. Very often, of course, the nature of the child's responses is such that one gets only a tentative or approximate threshold measurement, but even this is of extreme clinical value, since it enables one to say that hearing is no worse than a given figure, or to note that responses are made at a given intensity level. The results of speech audiometry may be expressed directly in decibel units, which become a direct measure of how the child being tested compares to the normal-hearing youngster.

OTHER TESTING METHODS

It is evident from the preceding description of pure tone and speech audiometry that a very accurate idea of a child's hearing ability can be derived from tests of this sort, provided he is capable of understanding what he is to do and is willing and able to cooperate with the audiometrist. There remain, however, large numbers of children who, by reason of age or some other factor, simply cannot be given routine audiometric examinations with any expectation of success. Clinically, the estimation of the hearing status of such children is of extreme importance for both medical and educational reasons. Although the problem of how to test such youngsters has received a great deal of attention in recent years, and several ingenious examination techniques have been worked out, much remains to be done before it will be possible to make entirely reliable and valid measurements of children of all ages and types. The parent and teacher should, of course, be familiar with the uses and limitations of these methods.

Psychogalvanic Skin Response Testing

In recent years there has been great interest in the adaptation of what is called the psychogalvanic skin response (PGSR) to the measurement of hearing in children and infants. The psychogalvanic skin response itself has been known to exist for many years, but attempts to employ this phenomenon for hearing measurement are relatively recent. The PGSR is a reduction in the resistance of the skin to the passage of an electric current which can be brought about by a mild electric shock (the Feré effect).

This change in the resistance of the skin can be detected by the use of what is called a Wheatstone bridge associated in a circuit with certain other instrumentation. Results can be recorded in various ways. At least one manufacturer has designed a single compact unit containing the necessary components for convenient clinical use.

The actual hearing test involves the establishing of what is called a *conditioned response*. Most readers will recall the classical experiments of Pavlov in which a dog's saliva is caused to flow by the sight of food. This reaction to the sight of food is called the *unconditioned response*. Pavlov demonstrated that if another stimulus, such as the ringing of a bell, is given under relatively strict conditions along with the presentation of food to the animal, the second stimulus alone will become effective in arousing the secretion of saliva. The response has become *conditioned* to a stimulus which originally would not have aroused this response.

In PGSR audiometry the lowered skin resistance is the unconditioned response which is elicited by administering a mild electric shock to the subject. This response is conditioned (if it is) by repeatedly presenting a tone at a standard interval before each shock. If the tone alone is subsequently found to cause the lowered skin resistance, it is concluded that the subject "hears" the tone, and his threshold may thus be charted theoretically on the basis of this involuntary response, without any understanding or effort on his part. If the response cannot be conditioned, this is taken as evidence of failure to hear. The usual procedure is to place the small electrodes, which are connected in the Wheatstone bridge circuit, to the palm and back of the hand, and to deliver the test tone from a pure tone audiometer through a conventional headphone.

This technique offers much promise for children who are difficult to test, but a great deal more research and experience will be needed before PGSR audiometry becomes a satisfactory clinical tool for widespread use. Although some discouraging reports have been made, it appears to be the general opinion of audiologists that this technique makes it possible for the clinician who has the requisite skill in interpretation to decide whether or not hearing exists and to locate at least approximately the maximum possible amount of loss which could be present in children whose response becomes conditioned. Just how much margin of error is present in the obtained thresholds is a matter on which there is some disagreement. The PGSR hearing test may be carried out with infants or with children too young to understand or cooperate in the commoner methods of audiometry. The principal limitations to PGSR audiometry center around certain theoretic questions regarding the phenomena of the conditioned response and of hearing, and the practical problems arising from interpreting the child's responses, securing tolerance of the apparatus and similar difficulties. There are always children who are too intractable to be tested in any way.

Additional Conditioning Techniques

The principles of conditioning have been adapted in several other ways to the measurement of hearing in children. Strictly speaking, the galvanic skin response is a *reflex,* but conditioning may take place with responses which are essentially voluntary. This fact has been used in devising the "peep show" technique for detecting hearing losses in children. The equipment for the peep show consists of a toy house into which the child can look through a small window. Placed before him is a button which is pressed to illuminate the interior of the house, whereupon the child sees an attractive and interesting picture. Head-phones connected to an audiometer are worn by the child. The audiometrist is able, by manipulating the necessary controls, to make it possible for the child to illuminate the house only while a tone is being heard or immediately thereafter. In this way some children rapidly discontinue efforts to light the house, except when a tone is heard. Others will only *tend* to do so. In either case, the youngster's behavior will give evidence as to whether or not he is actually responding to the test tone.

Another similar device was used earlier in England by the Ewings. Their arrangement was much the same, except that the play device used for conditioning consisted of a lighted electric train which could be made to emerge from a tunnel when the child pressed the button. Actually, lighting the house or starting the train in these tests is merely another way for the child to respond to the test tone, rather than by raising the hand or pressing the signal button. However, unconscious learning may take place in the peep show and in the test used by the Ewings. Other simpler procedures involving similar kinds of conditioning may be employed by having the child place a block in a box when he hears a tone, or engage in some other interesting activity. The utilization of play activities to secure the child's conscious or unconscious cooperation and interest is a valuable clinical tool, especially with children who cannot be handled readily otherwise. There have been some attempts to condition responses such as the eye wink, the pupilary reflex to light and others, but these methods have not come into clinical use. The use of electroencephalography (EEG) or "brain waves" for detecting responses to sound also has been ap-proached tentatively, but such techniques are not yet of estab-lished value for this purpose.

Estimating Hearing Loss by Observation

When more formal methods fail, there is always the possi-bility of reaching at least a gross evaluation of the child's hear-ing by observing his behavior in response to ordinary en-vironmental sounds, or in what might be called unstructured situations. Usually, judgments of this sort tell the examiner little more than whether the child seems to be totally unresponsive to sound, or whether he does seem to hear at least some sounds. Nevertheless, observations of this type are often of great value in making a tentative diagnosis, and they may be made cautiously and systematically. Naturally, every effort must be made to interpret the child's behavior perceptively.

The manner in which environmental sounds influence the behavior and total developmental growth of the child is a subject much too complex for elaboration in this discussion. Suffice it to say that the contact which sound provides between the infant and the world around him, both the sounds of language and others, plays an important role in shaping the child's emotional growth and personality structure; when he is deprived of this contact there is likely to be a pattern of behavior which reflects this lack. There are typical behavioral signs of hearing loss or deafness which may be considered as diagnostic signs of possible auditory defect.

The lack of language development at the normal age should arouse an immediate question about hearing, for reasons which are obvious. Earlier, a diminished amount of babbling, or the absence thereof, may reflect a sensory loss. It is usually said that a deaf baby will begin to babble or indulge in vocal play at approximately the normal time (perhaps as early as the second or third month), but that this will neither increase significantly in amount nor duration, presumably because the child who does not hear fails to get the self-stimulation which occurs in the normal infant. There are, of course, other reasons for failure to babble.

In early infancy inability to hear may show itself in certain characteristic ways. Ordinarily the baby will respond to loud sounds by crying, turning his head toward the source of the sound or ceasing momentarily whatever activity he may be engaged in; consistent failure to show these signs may arouse the suspicion of hearing loss. Other suspicious behavior should also be watched for, such as failure to awaken easily in the presence of noise.

As the child grows older he naturally comes to be responsive to sounds in familiar ways: he learns to come when he is called, his attention is attracted by the voices of playmates, he listens to the radio, and so on. Failure to exhibit such behavior can be observed by the perceptive parent; its absence should be thought of as a possible indication of hearing loss. The child with reduced auditory acuity comes quite naturally to place great reliance on what he sees. This may result in the development of a high degree of skill in unconscious lip reading, which can be detected if one notes the differences in the child's responses when he can and cannot see the speaker. Different responses to loud and weak sounds can sometimes be noted. An extended discussion of the behavioral patterns of the deaf child and of the differences among the deaf, emotionally disturbed, mentally defective and aphasic children has been prepared by Myklebust (see bibliography).

In attempting to measure the hearing of young children there are certain procedures which enable the examiner to observe the child's response to sound in at least a semicontrolled situation. These often prove very illuminating. One common technique is to create a loud sound outside the child's field of vision with the voice or some type of sound maker. The child without impaired audition will naturally turn to the source of the sound, give a startle response or react in some other appropriate manner. Sometimes one can thereby make at least gross judgments about the child who is suspected of having a hearing loss. Minimal clues may include such things as changes in facial expression, momentary cessation of activity, or some movement which could show that the child has heard. In all such "testing" one must be sure that the child is not reacting to a visual stimulus or to vibration. The deaf or hard of hearing child may become particularly sensitive to vibrations which are "felt" rather than heard. He might, for instance, enjoy music because he feels vibrations, or detect his father's footsteps on the front porch in the same way. At best, of course, this sort of clinical observation carries the great risk of misinterpretation, particularly when the child's responses are inconsistent, as they so typically may be; nevertheless, the behavioral signs are some-times unmistakable. The pure tone and speech audiometers may be used for these gross sound response tests. Occasionally the pure tone audiometer will demonstrate differential reactions to sounds of different frequencies in this kind of observation. Noise making toys which create sounds of different pitches, such as horns, whistles, "snappers," and so on, may be used. The experienced observer can sometimes make a surprisingly accurate judgment of the intensity of the sound to which the child responds.

It is hoped that the preceding discussion will serve as a basis for understanding the problems involved in measuring the hearing of the young child. If this has been the case, parents and teachers should now know when children under their care have had the best possible hearing diagnosis at the outset, and if the continuing evaluation of hearing ability is adequate as medical treatment and educational training are instituted.

The following bibliography provides sources of additional and more detailed information on the measurement of hearing.

BIBLIOGRAPHY

BLOOMER, H.: A simple method for testing the hearing of small children. J. Speech Disorders 7:311–312, 1942.

BUNCH, D. C.: Clinical Audiometry. St. Louis, C. V. Mosby, 1943.

DAHL, LORAINE A.: Public School Audiometry. Danville, Illinois, The Interstate Publishers and Printers, 1949.

DAVIS, H.: Hearing and Deafness: A Guide for Laymen. New York, Murray Hill Books, 1947.

DIX, M. R. AND HALLPIKE, C. S.: The peep show: A new technique for pure tone audiometry in young children. Brit. Med. J. 2:719–731, 1947.

EWING, IRENE R. AND A.W.G.: Speech and the Deaf Child. Washington, D. C., The Volta Bureau, 1953.

FLETCHER, H.: Speech and Hearing. New York, D. Van Nostrand, 1929.

HARDY, W. G. AND BORDLEY, J. E.: Special techniques in testing the hearing of children. J. Speech & Hearing Disorders 16:122–131, 1951.

—— AND PAULS, MIRIAM: The test situation in PGSR audiometry. J. Speech & Hearing Disorders 17:13–24, 1952.

HIRSCH, IRA J.: The Measurement of Hearing. New York, McGraw-Hill, 1952.

KEASTER, J.: A quantitative way of testing the hearing of young children. J. Speech Disorders *12*:159–160, 1947.

MYKLEBUST, HELMER R.: Auditory Disorders in Children. New York, Grune & Stratton, 1954.

SALTZMAN, MAURICE: Clinical Audiology. New York, Grune & Stratton, 1949.

UTLEY, JEAN: What's Its Name? A Guide to Speech and Hearing Development. Urbana, Ilinois, University of Illinois Press, 1950.

WATSON, L. A. AND TOLAN, T.: Hearing Tests and Hearing Instruments. Baltimore, Williams & Wilkins, 1949.

WESTLAKE, HAROLD: Hearing acuity in young children. J. Speech Disorders 7:7–14, 1942.

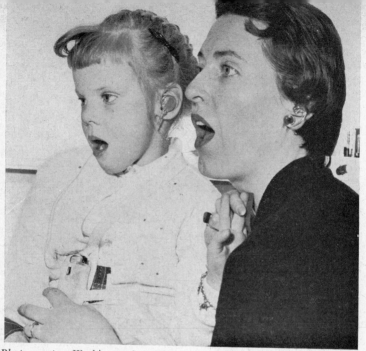

Photo courtesy Washington State Department of Health

5

Hearing‖Aids for Children

MECHANICAL HEARING DEVICES

THE purpose of a hearing aid is to amplify or increase the loudness of sound so that it can be heard more plainly or at greater distance. There are a number of ways of increasing the loudness of sound. One of the commonest ways is to collect more sound energy from the air than is normally collected by the listener's ear. Cupping the hand behind the ear is an age-old and still widely used method of increasing the amount of sound that reaches the ear. Ear trumpets and speaking tubes of all ages and descriptions are based on the principle of increasing the collection and delivery of sound energy to the ear. In addition

114

to the funnel effect of an ear trumpet, many devices utilize the principle of reaching out to catch the sound close to its source, thus reducing the scatter and waste of energy. The speaking tube illustrates both of these principles. It is designed with one small end to be inserted in a listener's ear while the other end is flared like a horn and intended to be held near the speaker's mouth. The effectiveness of this method of conserving sound energy may be demonstrated easily by connecting a small plastic funnel to a short piece of rubber tubing and talking through it. Except for the inconvenience and limited application of a speaking tube many hard of hearing persons would find such a device about as satisfactory as an electric hearing aid. For some elderly people whose main objective is to visit with one person at a time the speaking tube may actually seem more natural and pleasant than an electric amplifier. It is obvious that such a tube can be purchased cheaply or can be built at home at negligible cost. The speaking tube should be kept in mind particularly for those people who, because of age or eccentricity, are unable to cope with an electric instrument.

The physician's stethoscope is another application of the speaking-tube principle. A sensitive diaphragm is used as a probe near the source of the sound being studied, while rubber or plastic tubes channel the sound directly to the ears of the listener. It is indeed fortunate that many physicians who have suffered some loss of hearing acuity are able to hear and interpret effectively the signals carried by a stethoscope. Goldstein no doubt had in mind the design of a stethoscope when he devised the simplex hearing tube,[1] which was and still is used to deliver a strong binaural signal of speech or music to stimulate residual hearing in children.

Further illustration of improving the utilization of sound energy is seen in the use of a megaphone. By this mechanical means, sound energy can be directed to some extent toward a chosen area. It reduces the normal scatter of energy and delivers more sound to the place where it is wanted. A megaphone reversed, with the small end held to the ear, becomes, of course, an ear trumpet, and accordingly increases the collection of sound at the ear.

The importance of distance from the source of sound always should be borne in mind when there is a question regarding

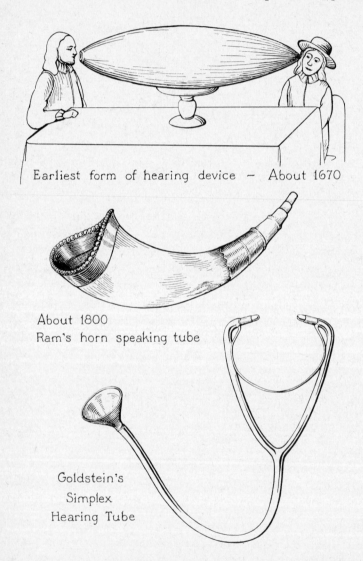

Earliest form of hearing device — About 1670

About 1800
Ram's horn speaking tube

Goldstein's
Simplex
Hearing Tube

(Used by permission The Laryngoscope Press, St. Louis. Redrawn by S. Risser)

acuity of hearing. Whether or not a hearing aid is being used, it is helpful for a speaker to be close to a listener who is hard of hearing. This becomes more apparent when we recall that the intensity of sound traveling in open air decreases in proportion to the square of the distance it travels. Everyone who associates with a hard of hearing person learns that close range conversation rather than use of loud voice usually is the key to comfortable understanding. With this in mind, parents, teachers and others who deal with hard of hearing children should remember the tremendous value of abundant talking, reading and singing in a clear, pleasant voice near the child's ear. We only have to note the loudness and the distance at which children with normal hearing listen to radio, phonograph or television in order to appreciate a child's taste for a strong auditory signal. We may note further that a child with mild impairment of the middle ear is inclined to adjust auditory volume to a level that drives adults to distraction, or from the room.

There have been a number of small prosthetic devices designed to fit entirely within the external ear and intended to increase the intensity of sound for the wearer. Probably the commonest of these is a moistened pellet of cotton for use in ears that have a perforated drum membrane or in which the drum membrane is absent entirely. The usual method of applying this type of prosthesis is to roll a wisp of cotton into a tiny tapered cylinder, moisten it with an inert oil and place the small end in contact with the stapes or the round window while the larger end occupies the space where the drum membrane should be. Although the number of cases in which this sort of aid proves worth while seems to be very limited, there is no doubt that some individuals have derived practical help from such a simple device. Obviously a moistened piece of cotton in the ear will not stay moist indefinitely, and it is likely to move from the effective location from time to time. Ordinarily it is advisable, if not essential, to have each application made by an experienced otologist. However, some patients have learned to apply a cotton prosthesis to their own ears effectively.

Another mechanical appliance that occasionally has proved beneficial to individuals whose middle ear mechanism has been damaged or destroyed is a small bristle attached to an artificial membrane. This device is applied and worn in much the same way as the cotton pellet. Like the cotton prosthesis, it is intended as a substitute for the normal drum membrane and ossicles. The artificial membrane is designed to span the external auditory canal so that it will catch the full impact of sound energy that enters the ear canal. The bristle extends from the central portion of the membrane across the middle ear to a sensitive point (probably the footplate of the stapes) on the wall of the inner ear. A sound-conducting apparatus similar to that found in certain lower animals is thereby constructed. While this mechanism would seem to have considerable merit from a theoretic standpoint, there is little evidence of its practical value. Apparently the problems of suitable placement, attachment and maintenance of the membrane and bristle challenge satisfactory solution. Effective application of such an apparatus is possibly even a more delicate maneuver than applying a cotton prosthesis properly. Accordingly, its use is very rare.

In assessing the value and importance of these mechanical type aids to hearing, it must be remembered that very few people present the precise conditions that make such aid feasible and practical. Furthermore, most individuals who do derive benefit from one of these devices very likely would get as much or more help from a conventional electric hearing aid.

QUACK HEARING DEVICES

It is not surprising that the production and sale of pseudo-scientific gadgets for the correction of hearing deficiencies has been and remains a tempting enterprise for unscrupulous promoters. It is logical that hard of hearing people as well as their relatives and friends find a strong appeal in any kind of small apparatus that fits inconspicuously within the ear and promises to be the complete solution to all hearing problems. One of our characteristics as human beings, and particularly as Americans, has been to believe in the seemingly impossible. Our technologic advances in recent years have been such as to expand continually our faith in scientific achievement. The modern electric hearing aid itself tends to prove that "miracles" may happen. Then the fact that simple mechanical devices like the ones described have been known occasionally to work gives credence to the possibility that a small miraculous appliance for improvement of hearing might be available. Following the real evidence at hand and the apparent logic of clever advertisements, even a thoroughly rational person is likely to wonder and ask: "Why not expect to find a hearing aid that can be worn entirely within the ear and have it provide satisfactory reception?"

This is a matter that calls for more than brief denunciation on the part of a physician or other counselor. A hard of hearing person or the parent of a child with impaired hearing is prone, in desperation, to grasp at any straw. The damage done by groping in the dark for some mysterious solution to a problem is not limited to waste of money. More important may be the wasted time and the disappointment that follows.

In view of the strong susceptibility of people in general and of hard of hearing people in particular to short-cut or novel means of alleviating a difficult situation, it is extremely unfortunate that no systematic approach has been employed in regulating the advertising and selling of hearing aids. Since regulation of the distribution of hearing aids does not appear to be forthcoming, it behooves every professional person responsible for advising those with hearing problems to know what can be done and what can *not* be done by a particular type of hearing device. And it is not enough that a counselor on hearing know the simple facts; he needs to know how to explain and demonstrate these facts to the patient or parent concerned.

ELECTRIC AMPLIFICATION

Although mechanical type hearing aids are of interest and warrant some consideration, they are relatively unimportant and ineffective in comparison to present-day electric amplifiers. With an electric amplifier we need not be so seriously concerned with conservation or collection of sound energy. The electric current or the batteries used provide an additional reservoir of power which can be converted into the desired sound pattern and delivered with relative efficiency to the listener.

An electric amplifier is most commonly exemplified by a telephone circuit or a public address system. Such a system is made up of three basic units: a microphone, an amplifier or booster circuit and a receiver or speaker. The microphone picks up sound waves from its environment and from this energy produces an electric current similar in pattern to that of the initiating sound. The amplifier draws on an electric line or a battery for power to increase the magnitude of the current supplied by the microphone. The receiver in turn converts the magnified electric current back into amplified sound waves. In a high fidelity system each of these units is so designed and so matched that the sound emitted from the receiver is essentially the same in pattern as that picked up by the microphone.

Essentially all amplifying systems are arranged so that the amount of amplification may be controlled by regulating the addition of power in the amplifying circuit. Amplifiers usually are arranged so that the power is controlled by a knob that may be turned up or down by the listener. This knob, of course, is the volume control which we find on public address systems, hearing aids, radios and essentially all audio-amplifying systems.

Aside from the volume control, some amplifiers have one or more additional switches that may be used to alter intentionally the pattern of sound that is transmitted. For certain listeners or for certain purposes it may be desirable to change the quality of sound from its original pattern so that some tones are emphasized more than others in the transmission. Within certain limits such changes can be effected and controlled by the amplifying system.

The limitations in control of tone quality and also in attainment of high fidelity reproduction are much greater in small hearing aids than in larger systems. Accordingly, it is to be expected that a stationary or desk model amplifier will give a stronger and clearer signal than will a wearable hearing aid. The size and quality of earphone used in a system are of particular importance in the attainment of high fidelity. The small button-type receiver used in most wearable hearing aids introduces distinct characteristics of its own into the sound that is delivered. These characteristics are likely to exert significant influence on the intelligibility of speech. Many hearing aid companies provide for selection among a variety of receivers depending on the type of hearing loss and the listening tastes of the wearer. Most stationary and semiportable type amplifiers use receivers that are approximately the size of the external ear. Receivers of this size and of high quality are capable of delivering very accurate reproduction of speech at high intensities.

Compression Amplification

In addition to the manual control of volume, some amplifying systems have provisions for automatic control of volume. That is to say, the excessively loud or strong sound waves going through the amplifier are made to exercise instantaneous control of the gain so that they limit the intensity of their own transmission. In such a system an unusually strong sound wave or intensity peak that might be amplified to the level of pain is made to limit itself to a prescribed maximal intensity so that the listener need not experience discomfort from sharp sound peaks even though the gain for most of the signal is as high as desirable. This type of limitation is called "compression amplification." It has the desirable feature of compressing the whole wave that is too loud in such a way that it approaches maintenance of the original wave form and thus retains most of the true characteristics of the signal.

Peak Clipping

Another way of limiting the ceiling of intensity is by peak clipping. Every amplifier has a maximal output, and if the stronger waves or peaks of a signal of variable intensity such as speech tend to exceed this maximum, they are automatically limited or clipped to the level that the instrument will carry. The design or adjustment of an amplifier may be such as to introduce this ceiling at whatever level is desired. If it is placed too low, the peak clipping process occurs excessively and the resultant signal becomes badly distorted. It is obvious that any peak clipping tends to distort the wave form, but a reasonable amount of it may be employed without a prohibitive effect on the intelligibility of speech. Application of peak clipping then becomes a matter for judicious compromise. A little of it may make amplified speech tolerable and therefore satisfactory to a particular individual, while too much of it may render the signal unintelligible and thus unsatisfactory.

Peak clipping has the advantage over compression amplification of being more simply and inexpensively applied. Accordingly, it is being provided in some wearable hearing aids, while compression amplification has been available so far only in larger amplifying systems.

Vacuum Tube Hearing Aids

The vast majority of hearing aids in current use are vacuum tube instruments that are small enough to be worn by a person with only moderate inconvenience. These instruments normally consist of a microphone, a battery-powered amplifier and a receiver. The microphone, the transmitter, and the batteries usually are built in a single case that approximates the size of a package of cigarets and weighs from five to ten ounces. The exact size and weight vary somewhat with the make and model of instrument. Most hearing aid receivers in current use are button-like units approximately one-fourth of an inch thick with a diameter comparable to that of a nickel. They are attached to the amplifier by a thin electric cord and are intended to be worn in the external ear by attachment to an individually molded earpiece. A very small minority of hearing aid wearers use a bone conduction vibrator in place of the type of receiver just described. These units approximate the size and shape of the end of a man's thumb from the first joint and are intended to be held firmly against the bone behind the ear by use of a headband.

Most hearing aid amplifiers operate on two small batteries which are designated the "A" battery and the "B" battery. The "A" battery provides current to heat the filament of a vacuum tube, thereby releasing electrons or negative charges which flow through a gate or grid to the plate of the tube where they initiate the output current. The "B" battery maintains a positive charge on the plate to attract the free electrons. It also is connected in circuit with the receiver through which it drives the output current. The input current from the microphone is delivered to the grid which acts as a gate or valve regulating the flow of electrons between the filament and the plate. When the charge on the grid is relatively negative, it will tend to repel or block the flow of electrons. When the grid is less negative, it permits more current to flow through this gate. Thus, the relatively strong current from the "B" battery is made to simulate the pattern of the relatively weak current from the microphone. This pattern is established by the impinging sound waves. The receiver converts the output current back into sound waves which are similar in pattern but stronger than the waves that struck the microphone initially. Because of the nature of this governing process, the vacuum tube is called appropriately an "electronic valve" and is the basic principle on which most present-day audio-electric instruments are built.

Most hearing aids of average power output use three vacuum tubes and have relatively complex circuits that include other parts such as transformers, condensers, resistors and controls of various kinds. These additions and complications do not alter the basic principle illustrated by the one-tube amplifier. For the present purpose there is no need to explore the intricacies of hearing aid circuits. The operator or person directing the operation of a hearing aid need not feel responsible for understanding details of design or of intricate repair. It is helpful, however, for him to understand the basic principles of amplification and it is imperative that he become familiar with the various controls and adjustments on the instrument or instruments he expects to use.

Volume Controls

The commonest arrangement on hearing aids is to combine the off–on switch with the volume control. After the volume is reduced the maximal amount, an additional turn of the control causes a click that breaks the circuit and turns off the instrument. With this switch off, there is no drain on either battery. However, as an added precaution against waste of power and possible damage from battery acids, most manufacturers of hearing aids advise removal of one or both batteries when the instrument is not in use. A few instruments will be found that provide an off–on switch that is independent of the volume control. This arrangement has the advantage of permitting the volume setting to be left stationary when the instrument is turned off, thus avoiding readjustment of the volume each time it is worn. It has the disadvantage of presenting more controls for the wearer to manipulate.

In addition to the external volume control, a number of hearing aids have a switch somewhere inside the case that permits selection of either high or low gain. On some instruments the adjustment of this switch is comparable to the basic selection of a high-powered or a low-powered instrument. On others, the difference between high and low gain is relatively slight. The selection of magnitude of gain, like the selection of instrument size and battery voltage, depends primarily on the degree of hearing loss, but also may be related to the type of impairment and even to some extent to the auditory taste of the individual.

The lack of uniformity from instrument to instrument in providing for selection of gain characteristics can be overcome only through familiarity with the adjustments and characteristics of each instrument under consideration. Most of the leading manufacturers of hearing aids provide either different models or an adjustment for a substantial change in gain to accommodate wearers needing either a moderate or a high degree of amplification.

Another control that is becoming commoner on hearing aids is one that regulates the maximal output of the instrument. As more gain in volume has been made possible by improved tubes and circuits, it has become increasingly important to limit the intensity of sound peaks for some wearers. This ceiling limita-

tion has been applied in a variety of ways, ranging from mechanical obstructors in the receiver openings to peak clipping
devices in the amplifying circuit. This type of control differs
from regulating the gain characteristics of an instrument in that
it is independent of the input signal. Even though a signal at
the microphone be extremely loud and the gain of the amplifier
relatively high, a limiting valve may be employed to keep the
maximal output to a level that is tolerable to the wearer.

The knowledge of whether or not an instrument has a limiting control on the output and the method of operating this
control must be gained from the descriptive literature or from
demonstration of a particular instrument. To date, there has
been no uniformity in provision for, or arrangement of, an output control in the various brands or even in various models of
a given brand of hearing aid.

TONE CONTROLS

Most hearing aids have a tone control that adjusts the relative strength of the high-frequency, low-frequency and middle-
frequency tones that are amplified. Emphasis on one or another
tonal range usually is achieved by a combination of condensers
and resistors in the circuit that transmits one range of tone more
efficiently than another. The process actually is that of suppress-
ing the undesired range while the tones to be emphasized are
transmitted relatively more efficiently.

A number of manufacturers place the tone control inside the
case with the intention that it be adjusted only by the sales representative. In some instances a special tool is required to make
the adjustments. However, the commoner arrangement is to
place the tone control switch outside the case and to label the
positions in a simple manner so that the wearer can select or
change the tone emphasis as desired.

The advantages and disadvantages of each of these arrangements are obvious. On the one hand, it is judged that the selection of tone emphasis can be made best by the hearing aid
representative who has had experience with the particular instrument and with the results other wearers have had with it.

It is believed by some designers that the process of trial and experimentation with the tone control is confusing to the wearer, and that it merely aggravates the difficulties of learning to use an instrument. On the other hand, it is felt by many designers that each wearer is best qualified to judge the tone emphasis that suits him. Those who make the tone control readily accessible also feel that the wearer may want to change the tone adjustment according to the listening situation.

A few instruments of recent design have entirely eliminated the tone control. This action is based on the reasoning that the best tone pattern for most wearers is one that approaches as nearly as possible high fidelity reproduction. Accordingly, certain instruments have been built with only one control, that being the combined off–on switch and volume control.

At the opposite extreme from the manufacturers who build hearing aids with no choice of tone emphasis are those who claim to do "prescription fitting." This refers to the claim or implication that each hearing aid is built or adjusted uniquely to meet the specific needs of the person who is to wear it. In some instances the "fitting" is done at the time the instrument is being assembled at the factory. More commonly, it is done by the sales representative who selects and manipulates tube combinations, tone controls and receiver characteristics according to the needs of the individual to be "fitted." While some of the efforts toward precise individual fitting of hearing aids are noteworthy, it is doubtful whether the full advantages implied by "prescription fitting" have often been achieved. There are at least two serious limitations in the attainment of exact fitting with a wearable hearing aid. In the first place, it is doubtful whether it can be determined without thorough and prolonged study just what tone pattern is best for a given individual. In the second place, the technical possibilities of delivering a prescribed tone pattern with a standard-sized hearing aid are strictly limited.

This reservation regarding the merits of "prescription fitting" is not meant to detract from the value of careful selection of tone and volume adjustments which are provided on many hearing aids. It is clear to everyone who has dealt with the trial and evaluation of hearing aids that certain tone patterns do suit a given individual better than other patterns, and also that an individual may interpret the speech he hears with one adjustment better than with another. There is no doubt either that many experienced and responsible hearing aid representatives are highly skilled in helping the wearers of their apparatus to select the adjustments that are suitable for them. But again, we should bear in mind that most selections of components and adjustments in hearing aids are made on the basis of relative values and on subjective judgments rather than on precise measurements.

Transistor Hearing Aids

Since the advent of transistors in the construction of hearing aids this type of instrument has essentially replaced vacuum-tube amplifiers in wearable hearing aids. Most of the technical difficulties that were encountered during the initial use of transistors have been resolved so that they now meet all the requirements of wearable hearing aids. Transistors are small crystal units made at present from a rare element known as germanium. This material has the unusual property of allowing an abundant flow of electrons from a relatively minute electric current. The pattern of this flow can be controlled by the input current from a microphone. Thus, the transistor instrument performs the same basic valve action as does the vacuum tube.

Since there is little or no waste of current in production of heat and light in the transistor, it has proved to be remarkably more efficient in battery consumption than are vacuum tubes, which dissipate much of the current supplied them in heat and light energy. Only one battery is required to operate a transistor hearing aid. The exact voltage and size of batteries vary from instrument to instrument, but in general the battery compares to the "A" battery in vacuum-tube sets and lasts much longer than a battery of comparable size in vacuum-tube instruments. From this, it is apparent that the cost of batteries for operating a transistor hearing aid should be only a fraction (possibly as little as one tenth) of that for operating the average vacuum tube set.

In addition to the economy of operation, transistors have been reported to be unusually durable. Their simplicity and the absence of heat generation suggest that they may be considerably more rugged than vacuum tubes, which represent a rather delicate assembly of metal and glass and which must burn out eventually from the heat generated in the filament. Although some of the early expectations as to the durability of transistors were slow in materializing, there is no question now that they will stand up under actual wearing conditions.

The use of transistors in hearing aids has brought about a substantial reduction in the size of instruments. This in turn has made it possible to wear the aids on the head in a number of ways. Some instruments are pinned in the hair, while others hang back of the ear and are held in place by a semirigid cord or tube that extends around the auricle into the concha of the ear. Certain of the smallest instruments are held partially in the canal and concha of the ear with varying amounts of protrusion from the ear. At the time of this writing the commonest way to wear hearing aids on the head is to attach them in some way to the frames of eyeglasses. There has been an almost continuous modification of design and reduction in size of these latter hearing aids so that many of the current models add very little in size or appearance to the average plastic frames of glasses.

The construction of an entire hearing aid in one bow of eyeglasses and of small instruments that can be worn in or behind one ear has greatly advanced the practicality of using binaural amplification. Until recently the use of a hearing aid in each ear was a rare occurrence. Whatever theoretic advantages this offered were offset by practical and technical difficulties. Most of those who did attempt to achieve binaural amplification did so by attaching two receivers to a single amplifier. This does not provide all of the features of true binaural hearing. As hearing aids have been made smaller and designed to wear at or near the ear to which the sound is delivered, true binaural amplification has become practicable.

Certain limitations in the amount of gain that can be achieved without feedback are inherent in wearing a hearing aid near the ear it serves. In every amplifying system there must be some separation or acoustic insulation between the microphone and the speaker to avoid acoustic feedback. The greater the amplification that is desired the greater must be the insulation between the units. Thus it is apparent that very tiny instruments in which the microphone and receiver are closely coupled must be limited in acoustic gain. Despite this limitation the benefits of wearing small hearing aids on the head have been significant. No doubt this is due partly to the elimination of noises that are produced by the friction of clothing when instruments are worn on the body. Also there seems to be better reception of sound from all directions and better localization of sound when the microphone is worn on the head. The ability to localize sound may be enhanced further by the use of an instrument in each ear.

Binaural Hearing Aids

A full evaluation and complete understanding of all the factors involved in binaural amplification has not been achieved. There has been relatively little objective research on which to base judgments regarding the use of two hearing aids. From the subjective point of view there have been numerous and impressive reports in favor of wearing a hearing aid in each ear. On theoretic grounds the merits of binaural amplification are indisputable. Among the advantages that are attributed to binaural hearing aids are improved fidelity of sound, better discrimination of speech, greater ease of listening and improved ability to locate the source of sound. These improvements may help toward restoring the capacity to listen selectively to one of several sounds in the environment. Since this function of hearing appears to be of signal importance in the process of communication, any gain in this direction is worthy of attainment. There is little doubt that binaural amplification offers a way for many people to hear more clearly and to communicate more satisfactorily than they could otherwise do. However, not all of the evidence points toward the use of two hearing aids by every hard of hearing person. If there were no other deterrents, the cost of two instruments would prevent many people from purchasing and maintaining two aids. The retail price of hearing

aids has been held absurdly out of proportion to the cost of production and to the price of other prostheses, such as eyeglasses
and braces. Many people find it a genuine hardship to buy and
maintain even one hearing aid. Other practical considerations
may be at variance with the theoretic conclusions regarding
binaural amplification. Some individuals simply do not like a
hearing aid in each ear. Unless the advantages can be clearly
demonstrated, they will not pay the price and take the trouble
to wear two aids. Such demonstration is by no means a certainty.
There are hearing conditions which result in significantly
poorer hearing with two aids than with one. This is most
apparent in cases where one ear suffers decidedly more recruitment and distortion than the other.

It would seem that the application of binaural amplification
should be based on individual considerations and that theoretic
benefits should be reconciled with demonstrable results as well
as subjective impressions.

Undoubtedly, further research and development in the performance of transistor hearing aids will be intensive in the immediate future. It is inevitable that the status of hearing aids
will change, possibly to a very significant degree, between the
time of this writing and the time it reaches its first readers. Possibly the only reliable counsel to give regarding hearing aids of
the future is that those professionally concerned with the evaluation and selection of instruments must accept the responsibility
of keeping themselves informed on changes and developments
in the field.

Receivers for Wearable Hearing Aids

As mentioned earlier, an integral part of every hearing aid is
the speaker or, as it is more commonly called, the receiver. In a
sense the receiver is the most important part of any sound-re-
producing system since it is the unit that converts the amplified
electric current back into a pressure pattern of sound waves. It
is this pressure pattern of physical energy that stimulates the
auditory mechanism rather than any electric phenomena occurring between the instrument and the ear or the nerves. This

point bears emphasis since many people make inquiries which indicate that they have been led or allowed to believe that a hearing aid can stimulate the nervous system in some way independently of the function of the ears. It was mentioned also that receivers introduce one of the most serious limiting features of most wearable hearing aids. The necessity, or at least the high desirability, of smallness in hearing aid receivers has posed one of the most difficult problems for hearing aid engineers. The engineers and the hearing aid industry have met this challenge remarkably well, and there is a prospect of continued progress in the quality and performance of hearing aid receivers.

Air Conduction Receivers

The vast majority (probably more than 95 per cent) of hearing aid receivers in use are so-called air conduction receivers. They are designated as such simply to distinguish them from bone conduction receivers, which serve a somewhat different purpose. The function of air conduction receivers in hearing aids is identical to that of earphones used in telephones, radios and all sorts of sound systems. It is comparable also to the function of loudspeakers, the difference being simply in the size of the vibrating diaphragm, and thus in the amount of air set into vibration. To state that function once again—it is that of utilizing the electric current from a transmitter to oscillate a diaphragm, which in turn sets the surrounding air into a vibratory motion which is sound.

Crystal Receivers. At present there are two principal types of air conduction receivers that have proved adaptable to use in wearable hearing aids. The crystal type of receiver was used widely for many years and may still be selected for some particular purpose. Its operation is similar to the reverse process of a crystal microphone. When the ouput current from an amplifier is applied to opposite sides of a crystal, the crystal bends in proportion to the voltage applied. A diaphragm is attached to the crystal in such a way that it responds to the bending motion. This movement of the diaphragm sets up sound waves in the surrounding air. This type of receiver inevitably introduces certain individual response characteristics which make it difficult to approach high fidelity reproduction and which also complicate the process of controlling the tone emphasis. With careful selection of crystals and appropriate matching of amplifier and receiver, the quality and emphasis of tone delivery can be regulated to some degree. Most wearable hearing aids that were sold a few years ago and a few now being sold employ crystal receivers effectively.

Magnetic Receivers. The commoner type of receiver found in current models of wearable hearing aids is a magnetic receiver. This type of receiver performs exactly the same function as that of a crystal receiver. The difference in the two types occurs in the principle of operation and in the tone characteristics. A magnetic receiver has a thin diaphragm of magnetic material mounted close to a permanent magnet. The drawing and repelling power of the magnet is altered by the strength and direction of the electric current from the amplifier passing through wire coils which are attached to the magnet. As the magnet pulls and repels the diaphragm, a vibratory motion is set up which produces sound waves in the surrounding air.

It has been possible to build magnetic receivers closer to specified standards than those attainable with crystal receivers. Magnetic receivers also have proved capable of reproducing a wider range of tones than most crystal receivers and in general they have less tendency to produce excessive emphasis or peaks in the tone pattern. This makes it possible to approach high fidelity reproduction more closely with magnetic than with crystal receivers. Accordingly, the magnetic type unit has come into use with most of the wearable hearing aids currently on the market.

Bone Conduction Receivers

Still another type of receiver is available with some instruments and is used effectively by a limited number of wearers. It is called a "bone conduction receiver" because it is designed to fit firmly on the mastoid bone behind the ear and to produce

vibration of the whole bony structure of the ear. The requirement of firm contact between the vibrating unit and the skin
covering the mastoid bone has made the use of a spring steel
headband essential for effective operation of bone conduction
receivers. All bone conduction receivers, like all air conduction
receivers, require an electric cord to carry the output current
from the amplifier to the receiving unit.

Most bone conduction vibrators operate on the principle of a
magnetic receiver, but are constructed in such a way that the
main force of the vibration is applied to a relatively heavy plate,
which makes up the face of the bone conduction unit, rather
than to the surrounding air. It is apparent and inevitable that
air or any substance in contact with the vibrating plate will be
set in motion to some extent, but the process is grossly inefficient
as compared to the relatively free motion of a thin diaphragm
in the air. Accordingly, if a vibrating bone conduction unit were
held close but not in contact with a normal ear, the sound very
likely would be heard softly but with only a fraction of the loudness that would be produced by the same energy applied through
an air conduction receiver. This gives a significant clue to the
relative efficiency of air conduction and bone conduction units.
It is apparent that a great deal more energy is required to drive
the relatively heavy plate which constitutes the face of a bone
conduction unit than to vibrate the thin, light diaphragm of an
air conduction receiver. Also, because of the relatively heavy
construction of bone conduction units, as well as the transmission characteristics of the skin and bones of the skull, it is difficult to transmit the higher pitched elements of speech by the use
of bone conduction receivers.

The matter of when it is possible and advisable to use a bone
conduction receiver will be dealt with in connection with the
selection of hearing aids. Suffice it here to note that the relative
inefficiency of bone conduction as compared to air conduction
has prompted many manufacturers to dispense with bone conduction models entirely, and those who do provide them sell
decidedly fewer bone conduction than air conduction units.

Permanent Molded Earpieces

An essential link in the transmission of sound from an air conduction receiver to the ear is the earpiece or the mold that holds the receiver in place. The earpiece usually is made from a hard transparent plastic compound, although for one reason or another it may be colored or may be made from some other material. For individuals who demonstrate an allergy to the customary compound, a hard rubber or some other substance may be employed. Various forms of sponge rubber and flexible plastic compounds are used also, particularly for tips or caps for more rigid molds and for tubes employed to extend the distance between the placement of the receiver and the wearer's ear.

Earpieces that are worn permanently or for any considerable time should be molded individually to fit the ear of the wearer. The fitting is usually made by insertion of a highly malleable substance that takes the form of the external ear and canal easily and then hardens quickly so that it may be removed without inconvenience or delay. This impression or cast is sent to one of a number of laboratories that specialize in making permanent earpieces patterned from the individual impressions. The finished earpiece must be built with a coupling snap and an open canal that leads from the coupling point down into the wearer's ear canal. Essentially, all air conduction receivers are made with a standard coupling arrangement at the opening where sound is emitted. A standard spring snap that attaches tightly to the coupling unit of the receiver is then added. An acoustic seal or sound-tight connection is desirable at this coupling.

Another important requirement of the earpiece is that it fit the ear and the ear canal comfortably and at the same time tightly enough to produce a good acoustic seal. If the earpiece does not fit properly either in the ear or at its junction with the receiver, there is likely to be leakage of sound which may produce a feedback or shrill squeal from the instrument. The presence of such a squeal is usually unpleasant to the wearer and to those around him. It also interferes with effective transmission of other signals. While there has been some dispute about the exact specifications of the most desirable earpiece, there is general agreement that it should carry a speech signal without serious distortion or marked reduction of power. It is generally agreed too that this can be done best with the standard type earpiece that holds the receiver close within the external ear and provides a relatively large air channel between the receiver and the ear canal. Any type of extension tube or molded fitting that permits the receiver to be worn away from the ear may be expected to sacrifice some degree of efficiency. The longer the tube the greater will be the distortion and loss of power. Accordingly, it is best to advise all those who wear or plan to wear hearing aids to forego the temptation to ask for or accept any of the so-called secret ear or hidden hearing devices that are designed to camouflage the wearing of a hearing aid.

TEMPORARY MOLDED EARPIECES

One of the problems that arise in an attempt to make a clinical evaluation or selection of hearing aids is that of providing a suitable earpiece for use in the trial of instruments. The point has been made frequently that the only proper way to try a hearing aid is with an individually molded earpiece. While there is little room for argument with this principle, the fact must be recognized that in a clinical situation it is often impractical to obtain a permanent custom-fitted earpiece in advance of the trial of hearing aids.

One approach to the problem is simply that of allowing enough time for an impression of the ear to be made and sent to one of the ear mold laboratories and for the finished earpiece to be returned before any trial procedures are undertaken. The time required for this action will vary, of course, with the relative locations of the clinic and the ear mold laboratory. At best, it is likely to take a day or two. Frequently, this delay is an inconvenience, and sometimes it prohibits the entire procedure.

Another possibility is for the hearing aid clinic to be equipped for the whole process of making the finished earpieces. Such a procedure requires a certain amount of special equipment and takes considerable time on the part of a technician. Again, there is the matter of some delay although it is not likely to be so long as when the impression is sent away to an ear mold laboratory. If circumstances warrant it, this probably is the most satisfactory arrangement.

A third method is to use dental wax as a fitting material over the stock inserts. A wide variety of sizes and shapes of the stock lucite inserts may be maintained. After an examination of the ear to be fitted, an insert is selected which as nearly as possible approaches the proportions and configurations of the ear. Then a coating of warm dental wax is applied over the insert, and while the wax is in a malleable state, it is pressed into the ear. The softened wax takes the shape of the concha of the ear and at the same time adheres to the surface of the lucite plug. This procedure provides very simply and quickly an individually fitted earpiece that is adequate for temporary purposes.

Group Hearing Aids

There are a number of stationary and nonwearable type instruments that must be taken into account in any consideration of hearing aids for children. Probably the commonest of these are group hearing aids which are designed for use in classrooms and gatherings of various kinds where several people wish to listen to the same amplified signal. These instruments are made up of one or more microphones, an amplifier that operates from an electric power line and a series of earphones or headsets. Occasionally, a loudspeaker is provided as an alternate unit in the system. There is usually a master control of volume or power and one or more tone controls on the amplifier. In the more modern and elaborate systems there may be provision for automatic volume control by means of peak clipping or by compression amplification. On most group hearing aids each set of earphones has an individual volume control. This permits each listener in a group to adjust the intensity to his particular need or taste while they all listen to the same speaker. On some instruments equipped with binaural earphones for each listener, it is possible to adjust for a stronger signal in one ear than the other. Systems of this basic type are provided with a wide variety of characteristics and adjustment features. Many such systems have been built to custom specifications. Many more have been assembled in "homemade" fashion by individuals and institutions. It is not at all uncommon to find some principal or electrician or a teacher of a school for the deaf who has selected, bought and assembled parts to provide his school with group hearing aids. As a result of "everybody getting into the act" it is almost impossible to compare one system with another. In general, it may be expected that the group hearing aids used in schools for the deaf and hard of hearing are capable of delivering sufficiently loud and reasonably clear speech signals to the wearers. As noted earlier, it is not too difficult a matter to reproduce and amplify speech highly and with reasonable fidelity by means of a large amplifier that draws abundant current from a power line and is matched to good quality microphones and earphones.

Probably the most significant and intensive use of group hearing aids is that carried on by schools, classes and clinics for the acoustically handicapped. In addition to the use of group hearing aids in schools, however, they are used extensively in churches, theaters, clubs and meeting places of all kinds.

AUDITORY TRAINING UNITS

Another type of amplifying unit that is gaining importance in the field of stationary hearing aids is what is called an "auditory training unit." Such a unit has much in common with a group hearing aid but is designated separately because of a number of features that are not found in most group systems. In addition to the usual microphone, amplifier and headset combination, it usually includes a record playing unit, a loudspeaker and either a radio or an attachment for an independent radio or television set. Most auditory training units are designed for use with one individual or for a small group of listeners. The manufacturers of these units have placed a premium on high intensity and high quality reproduction of sound. Many of these instruments have provision for automatic volume control which permits a high level of gain for the major part of a signal and at the same time puts a ceiling or a limiting valve on the more intense peaks in the signal. This feature in an amplifier makes it possible to operate the system at a higher intensity level without much danger of feedback or of reaching the listener's level of discomfort. Along with the high quality of amplification, the other desirable features of auditory training units are apparent. They permit convenient listening to the "live" voice, records, radio or television at high intensities without disturbing other persons in the environment. They also serve appropriately as public address systems if the loudspeaker is attached.

DESK HEARING AIDS

There is still another class of hearing aids that warrants consideration for children. They are commonly known as "desk" or "table model" aids. Their weight and construction are usually such as to make them portable, but not wearable. These instruments are intended for one listener only. They have the usual components of a microphone, an amplifier and a headset that may consist of either a single earphone or double earphones. The majority of instruments of this type require connection to an electric outlet as their source of power. However, some are designed to operate on batteries comparable to those used in portable radios. The relative convenience of each of these arrangements is obvious. An instrument powered by batteries can be carried and used anywhere while one without batteries must be stationed within the length of an extension cord from an electric outlet. On the other hand, an instrument with batteries requires occasional checking and changing of batteries, which entail some inconvenience and expense.

It would be reasonable to expect a higher potential gain and better control of tone quality from an instrument that draws its power from an electric outlet than from a battery set. To some extent this may be the case, but the difference in this respect among at least some of the instruments available is not impressive. Both the battery and the power line models may be equipped with high quality microphones, efficient earphones and other components large enough to permit high gain and adequate reproduction of speech signals.

Instruments of this type are used commonly and appropriately by elderly people who cannot be, or do not desire to be, active, and by business and professional people who find them suitable for office communication. They also can be used effectively with children for individual supervised auditory training and for building speech and language concepts. Frequently they are suggested for use at home with young acoustically handicapped children who are not ready to wear and manipulate hearing aids by themselves.

EVALUATION OF HEARING AIDS FOR CHILDREN

The evaluation of a hearing aid for a child may be a simple task that can be performed in an hour, or it may be a difficult matter that requires literally months or years of trial and observation. By evaluation here I am referring to an assessment of whether or not a hearing aid is worth while rather than to the relative suitability of different instruments.

Owing to improved instruments and procedures developed in recent years, it is possible to make reasonably accurate measurements of hearing on many children who could not have been tested satisfactorily some years ago. The more accurate the hearing tests, the more reliable will be the judgment on the value of a hearing aid. In general, children five years of age and older with normal mental and emotional capacity can be tested in somewhat the same way that adults are tested. That is, an audiogram can be made from voluntary responses to the tones presented, and tests of speech reception can be applied within the limits of the child's comprehension of language.

Hearing tests as applied to adults should always be briefed, modified, and motivated according to the age and maturity of a particular child. The usual classroom and clinical techniques of having a child carry on directed activity with objects and pictures can be adapted in evaluating his hearing either with or without amplification. Modern instruments and facilities of hearing clinics make possible more meaningful quantification of the results of such procedures. With very young children who do not respond voluntarily to speech or to tone signals, it may prove helpful to employ a conditioning process along with a skin galvanometer to detect involuntary responses to sound. A procedure known as psychogalvanic skin response audiometry has proved to be useful in evaluating the hearing of young children and even infants. Very briefly the procedure consists in conditioning a child to respond to sound as he normally does to an electric shock. This response manifests itself in a change of resistance in the skin to an electric current, and can be measured by a galvanometer attached to the skin (see page 107).

There are, of course, other means of observing involuntary responses to sound. The time-honored practices of watching a child's eyes, his facial expression, his head movements and his general activity must not be overlooked. These observations may tell us as much or even more than we learn from measuring skin resistance.

Ingenuity in motivating and guiding a child's interests and activities is probably the most valuable of all facilities in evaluating his hearing, or for that matter, any of his other capacities. No amount of instrumentation or design of material, valuable as they are, will substitute for a competent clinician's or teacher's skill in stimulating and directing a child's activity into meaningful patterns. In carrying out hearing tests, the activity may take many forms and involve many situations and kinds of materials. Noisemakers and toys of all sorts as well as real life objects such as water faucets, alarm clocks and musical instruments may be employed to stimulate a child's senses. Elaborate assemblies of instruments and materials, such as the Dix and Hallpike "peep show," [2] have been arranged for the purpose of making the observation of responses more reliable as well as more convenient. But despite all our efforts to examine and explore the hearing function thoroughly, in the case of some young, immature children, we must lean heavily on observable behavior and progress over a period of time to assess the value of a hearing aid. It may not be safe to pass judgment until the child has undergone supervision and training in the meaning of sound for as long as a year or more. On the other hand, with some children the evidence appears quickly, and we can demonstrate to our satisfaction during a single examination that a hearing aid is or is not appropriate.

In any judgment on the usefulness of hearing aids we must keep in mind the relative nature of the values. No person with a hearing loss can expect complete compensation by use of a hearing aid. In many instances the benefit falls far short of the goal. When this is the case, it presents a problem of weighing the degree of help against the cost and inconvenience of the instrument and any discomfort caused by it. So far as children are concerned, the factor of cost is modified by the existence of agencies that are willing to supply hearing aids to children whose parents cannot afford them. Although the inconvenience of wearable aids has been minimized in current models, it remains a factor of considerable concern to both children and adults. Nevertheless, the important considerations usually are reduced to those of benefit and comfort.

If we take note of the vast number of adults who distinctly need and do seek help from hearing aids, but who fail to get help or must forego the benefits because of discomfort, we should be more inclined to exercise caution in placing hearing aids on children. We are not justified in ignoring the complaints of real discomfort that are expressed by many children and adults alike as the result of subjection to amplification. On the other hand, we need not place undue importance on every displeasure that arises in adjusting to a hearing aid. Study of a child over a period of time and under appropriate circumstances will reveal the true state of affairs. Then efforts toward the proper solution can be directed accordingly.

Who Benefits From a Hearing Aid?

It is difficult to arrive at a set of criteria for recommending hearing aids even for adults and much more so for children. No hard and fast rules can be laid down for determining the need and suitability of an aid. Any set of standards must be tempered with good judgment and consideration of individual potentialities and limitations. Nevertheless, certain principles and guide-posts may be used in helping to determine who should wear a hearing aid.

In the case of adults, a general principle is that a hearing aid is appropriate for those with a permanent hearing loss of 35 decibels or more for the speech frequencies in the better ear. For children of school age this standard might suitably be lowered to 25 decibels since the need for serviceable hearing is particularly important for normal progress and development during the formal educative period. It is not likely that a great many preschool children will be found with permanent losses in the upper borderline area. However, every effort should be made to locate young children with auditory impairments before they show retardation in language and speech development. It is better to err in the direction of giving aid when it is not needed than to fail to give aid when it is needed.

With children, as with adults, the greatest degree of benefit and satisfaction from a hearing aid is likely to be experienced by those with losses for speech of 35 to 75 decibels. Children with losses in the speech range of 75 to 95 decibels usually require a period of supervised auditory training before the value of amplification can be determined. During this training period, one of the nonwearable type hearing aids is likely to be more suitable than a wearable instrument. Frequently, a period of auditory training will teach a child the significance of sound and create interest and pleasure in listening. When this is evident, it is appropriate to supply a wearable aid and teach him to use it.

If a thorough trial of amplification under supervision does not create interest in sound nor demonstrate benefit from it, or if the stimulation consistently causes discomfort to the child, it may be assumed that a hearing aid is not of practical value. Some children, like some adults, with losses of 75 to 95 decibels are unable to tolerate enough amplification to do them any good. If such is the case, it may be harmful not only physically but also psychologically to insist that they keep trying to use a hearing aid. A continual pressure on them to utilize their hearing in the face of an inability to do so is certain to cause frustration and promote or aggravate feelings of inadequacy.

Children with hearing losses greater than 95 decibels for the speech frequencies in the better ear, again like adults in the same category, cannot be expected to derive worth-while benefits from a hearing aid. Some awareness of sound may be gained by those of this group who can tolerate extremely high intensities, but its value for communication is negligible and accordingly is not usually considered justification for recommending use of an aid.

With children on whom we can obtain audiograms, the general principles regarding the shape of the curve may be applied. That is, a child with a flat audiogram or one in which the curve rises or falls gradually can expect good to excellent results from a hearing aid. Those whose audiograms show markedly falling curves, deep troughs, or other highly irregular patterns are likely to experience difficulty in understanding or learning speech from the sounds they perceive. These children, like those with severe degrees of loss, may never hear speech in the full pattern that normal ears perceive, but will still get enough from the rhythm and accent and the stronger components of speech patterns to help them immeasurably in the development of their own speech as well as in the understanding of the speech of others.

The Age for a Hearing Aid

The age and maturity of a child must be taken into consideration in assessing the value of a hearing aid. A distinction arises here between the use of wearable and nonwearable instruments and more particularly between independent use and supervised use of an aid. Any child known to have a hearing loss, but who demonstrates an awareness of sound and who can be stimulated pleasurably by loud sounds, is a candidate for supervised experience with amplification. It is obvious that these criteria are difficult to apply to babies, and accordingly it is well to forego the use of amplification until reliable professional assurance of the condition can be given.

A child should not be burdened with a wearable hearing aid until a reasonably accurate evaluation of his hearing is possible. This criterion properly places more importance on maturity and personality than on chronologic age. A further requirement related to age should be that the child understand the purpose of the aid and know how to manipulate it to fulfill that purpose. The child should be able to determine and to make known whether the stimulation from the instrument is pleasurable or uncomfortable. In the absence of this ability there is the danger, mentioned previously, of both physical discomfort and psychologic frustration.

The chronologic age and even the mental age at which children can meet these requirements will vary. Some children as young as two or three years of age may be able to wear hearing aids effectively if they have had the proper preparation and instruction. If a child has a practical degree of hearing at close range without amplification, the application of an aid may be primarily a matter of accepting the inconvenience of wearing it. In this event, a skillful parent or teacher may teach the child the purpose and the simple manipulations of an instrument at a very early age. More often than not a child will be four to six years old before he can be relied on to handle a wearable aid effectively.

At the same time that we caution against too early and thoughtless placing of wearable aids on children, we must warn against too much delay. Young children usually accept a hearing aid and adjust emotionally to it better than do older children. Adolescents in particular tend to experience pronounced and possibly prohibitive emotional trauma over the necessity of starting to wear such an appliance.

PRELIMINARY CONSIDERATIONS IN SELECTION OF HEARING AIDS

The number of hearing aid manufacturers and the variety of models are so great as to prohibit clinical consideration of each instrument. At the time of this writing there are more than fifty concerns in the United States producing hearing aids.

Each company puts out anywhere from one to a half dozen models simultaneously, and the models sometimes change within a six-month period. The result is a multitude of instruments far too great to be maintained by any one clinic. Each clinic faces the task of selecting a suitable number and quality of instruments for trial and demonstration purposes. A series of screening processes may be employed which will help limit both the number of instruments to be maintained by the clinic and the number to be considered for a particular individual.

Screening on the Basis of Manufacturing and Distribution Policies

The first screening is an obvious one based on practical considerations. It is impractical to maintain or recommend hearing aids which have no local representation. Both the clinic and the wearer would face the problem of inconvenience in service and repair in addition to the difficulty of the original procurement. In the larger communities there is sufficient representation among established concerns to afford an adequate stock and variety of instruments to choose from. In smaller communities it is wise to depend on the facilities of the nearest substantial city rather than limit the selection to strictly local agencies or to transient dealers.

The stability of both the manufacturer and the distributor is a significant criterion for selection of instruments. Certain companies have proved themselves to be dependable while others are questionable if not notably unreliable. Dependability may be judged somewhat on the basis of the soundness and reputation of the manufacturing concern, but one must also take into account distribution policies. In the event that an agent is known to have made frequent changes from one product to another or from one make of hearing aid to another, or if the agency for a given make of instrument changes hands periodically, it is justifiable to eliminate their instruments from consideration. If a particular dealer is deliberately antagonistic to the clinical service, it is of course injudicious to presume a working relationship. Such a situation frequently may be alleviated by appealing over the head of the uncooperative agent to a regional or central management.

A brief investigation will reveal important clues as to the responsibility that is borne by distributors for the performance of their instruments. In the matters of adjustment and service particularly, the local hearing aid representative has an opportunity to demonstrate the professional nature of his enterprise. If he accepts the challenge to render service with the same enthusiasm that he sells his product, he will welcome the cooperation of the hearing clinic. The agent who chooses to sell his hearing aids indiscriminately, avoiding all follow-up measures, will resent intrusion of the clinical service, so that cooperation is out of the question.

The whole matter of ethics and professional cooperativeness on the part of commercial hearing aid agencies creates a difficult situation to evaluate. At the same time, it is an essential basis on which to build an effective relationship among the hard of hearing patient, the hearing clinic and the hearing aid salesman.

Screening on the Basis of American Medical Association Acceptance

Another practical criterion on which the clinic may base selection of hearing aids is acceptance of the instruments by the Council on Physical Medicine and Rehabilitation of the American Medical Association. The Council arranges for detailed laboratory tests to evaluate the physical characteristics of each new make and model of instrument presented for approval. Only those aids which meet adequate standards of performance with regard to acoustic gain, frequency, response, distortion characteristics, noise level and battery drain are eligible for medical acceptance. All hearing aid manufacturers in the United States are privileged to submit their products for approval by the American Medical Association. If a company declines to apply for such approval or if the instruments submitted fail to meet the requirements, there is obvious reason to eliminate them from clinical consideration.

This limitation, applied in conjunction with that of responsible local representation and the elimination of obsolete models, provides a decided restriction in the number of aids to be dealt with clinically.

The criterion of acceptance by the American Medical Association needs to be applied with judicious leniency in the case of new model aids designed to replace formerly accepted models. Since it sometimes takes several months after a new model is in production for Council acceptance to be effected and reported, it is frequently justifiable to assume that approval will be granted. If a concern has customarily produced high grade hearing aids it is reasonable to expect that it would not supplant a Council-accepted model by one unsuitable for approval.

The hearing clinic must be constantly alert to the arrival of new instruments and must check Council reports regularly to be conversant with the status of available and approved equipment.

SCREENING ON THE BASIS OF HEARING LOSS AND THE KNOWN CHARACTERISTICS OF INSTRUMENTS

A final limitation of the number of hearing aids to be tried on a given individual may be made on the basis of the person's hearing loss and the physical characteristics of the instruments which have passed the previous screenings. Although complete data are not always available on the properties of the various aids, it is generally possible to combine the manufacturer's report and clinical experience to arrive at a practical estimate of the gross performance characteristics. It is hoped that the Council on Physical Medicine and Rehabilitation of the American Medical Association will institute the policy of making available, along with their general approval, the specific laboratory measurements of all hearing aids inspected. Such information would provide a basis for objective comparison of instruments and facilitate the clinical task of making preliminary selections.

It is generally conceded that exact fittings made on the basis of an audiogram and the laboratory performance of a hearing aid are unreliable in determining optimal hearing results. Still, a certain amount of theoretic selection is practicable. For example, certain instruments distinctly give a limited amount of amplification but have a relatively wide frequency response. Such an instrument obviously would be unsuitable for a person with severe hearing loss and lack of recruitment, but might afford ideal assistance for a subject with moderate impairment. Again, an instrument which produces unusually high gain at certain frequencies may be excluded in initial selection for a person with a low threshold for pain, or an instrument with peaked amplification at a relatively low frequency may be eliminated in choosing fittings for someone with a sharply declining audiogram curve.

Certain of the smaller instruments which for the sake of convenience use very small batteries and other components sacrifice some of the power and quality of amplification that are attainable in larger units. It is sometimes necessary to persuade a prospective hearing aid wearer that he must forego the convenience of a compact unit in order to obtain the desirable frequency response and margin in volume. However, this problem is becoming less acute with the employment of improved vacuum tubes and circuits, some of which provide adequate gain from low-voltage batteries. The advent of transistor instruments may further reduce the relationship between size of instrument and adequacy of gain.

CONSIDERATION OF COST AND CONVENIENCE

Ideally, the selection of hearing aids would be made on the basis of performance without regard to initial cost or expense of operation. Actually, many people in need of hearing aids must weight that need against the financial hardship of purchasing an instrument. In some cases the final decision of whether or not they will supply themselves with an instrument depends on the initial cost and estimated upkeep. Since standard model hearing aids vary in price from approximately $70 to $300, the prospective wearer is anxious to know what the differences are in cheap and expensive instruments. While the answer to this question cannot be a concise statement, the clinician can discuss with the subject some of the reasons for the range in cost and the differences in service customarily rendered by the various companies. Some of the differences are clearly explainable on the basis of distribution techniques and the amount of service afforded. Other differences are not apparent and must be assumed to be based on research and production costs and on business and profit policies of the different companies.

The relative costs and approximate life expectancy of different size and type batteries are important to a hearing aid user with limited means. He should be given information on the cost of batteries and on the approximate number of hours they are expected to operate with different aids. Estimates of these facts may be obtained from the manufacturers and checked with individual users and clinical experience. The established general principle is that smaller batteries cost more per unit of time than larger batteries. This principle clarifies the fact that the convenience of small, compact instruments must be paid for at least to some extent by greater operating expense. The whole perspective on battery costs and the relationship between these costs and the size of batteries used has undergone decided change wth the advent of transistor hearing aids. With a general knowledge of the situation regarding initial and operating cost of the various hearing aids, a person considering buying one is less likely to be disillusioned and more likely to choose one suitable to his needs and his means.

SELECTION OF HEARING AIDS FOR CHILDREN

So far as applicable, the selection of hearing aids for children should be based on the same principles as the selection of aids for adults. There will be of necessity many differences in procedures since children cannot be expected to participate in some of the comparative tests nor to exercise as accurate judgments as we ask of adults. Even with older children and thos with language facility, it is impractical to carry out some of the more lengthy procedures frequently used with adults. The goal is the same, however, in that we want to select an instrument that will deliver ordinary speech signals to the wearer as loudly as he wants them and with a quality of tone that is as pleasing as possible. We want to be sure that in the process of making average signals loud enough the instrument does not make strong signals painful to the wearer. In other words, the instrument should have a ceiling or limiting feature of some kind that is within the range of the wearer's tolerance. For adults and for children who can participate in speech reception tests, we want to find an instrument that gives speech as high intelligibility as possible and at the same time makes it sound natural and pleasant.

SELECTIVE AMPLIFICATION

The principle of selective amplification or of fitting a hearing aid to the audiogram in the sense of boosting each tone according to the amount of loss for that tone has been discarded to a large extent. However, the desirability or preference of a certain quality or tone emphasis is still recognized. For most hard of hearing persons the best understanding of speech is achieved either by high fidelity reproduction or by moderate suppression of the low tones which results in emphasis on the high tones. Since most instruments attempt to provide at least these two patterns of amplification, the choice between them usually is not of great concern.

SIGNIFICANCE OF THE AUDIOGRAM

Despite the trend away from selective amplification as a valid approach to the selection of hearing aids, the audiogram with both air conduction and bone conduction curves remains a measure of basic importance in recommending and choosing hearing aids. If obtainable, the audiogram tells approximately how much amplification should be provided. It shows the relative conditions of the two ears, and thus helps in determining the ear to be used. Comparison of air conduction and bone conduction thresholds indicates whether or not a bone conduction receiver should be considered. The audiogram reveals the presence of unusual patterns of hearing loss such as abruptly falling curves or highly irregular threshold contours. Knowledge of these conditions helps in anticipating the problems to be encountered with a hearing aid.

AIR CONDUCTION VERSUS BONE CONDUCTION

The question of whether to use an air conduction or a bone conduction hearing aid usually presents no serious problem. The vast majority of both children and adults will benefit more from air conduction than from bone conduction. If the diagnostic tests do not provide a clear indication of the preferable type of unit, trial performance with each type should differentiate between them.

Consideration of bone conduction may generally be limited to patients with pure conductive deafness or those whose ear condition prohibits use of an earpiece. Even among those with conductive deafness, many will hear better with air conduction receivers and therefore prefer them. Occasionally, some pathologic condition, such as malformation of the ears, may dictate the type of appliance that must be used.

In the event that the choice becomes optional, it should be remembered that air conduction receivers are basically more efficient than bone conduction units both in terms of frequency response and in utilization of power. As in other considerations, however, no wide generalization is warranted. It is essential to make each decision on the findings and results obtained.

WHICH EAR TO USE

The answer to the question of which ear to use with a hearing aid depends on medical findings, on relative acuity of the two ears and on certain practical considerations. If the medical report does not dictate the choice of ear for a hearing aid, the decision should be made on the basis of the relative acuity and the type of loss in each ear. In the absence of this information on children, we must again rely on trial and observation of results. So far as we are able to do so, we would advise a hearing aid for the ear that provides the best over-all hearing for speech. This goal is most often attained by using the aid in the better ear. In judging the better ear, we should consider not only the degree of loss but also the type of loss. If there is a difference in the type of loss in the two ears, it should be determined which ear tolerates amplification better and which is more efficient in perceiving speech. If the loss in both ears is less than 50 decibels, it may be advantageous to use the poorer ear, thus leaving the better ear unobstructed to the normal air-borne sounds. In this situation the sensitivity of the poorer ear is such that amplification should bring it up to a practical level, and the better ear has enough unaided sensitivity to be valuable without amplification. If the loss in the better ear exceeds 50 decibels or the loss in the poorer ear is greater than 60 decibels, it is generally advisable to fit the better ear. Under these conditions the chances are poor of aiding the severely impaired ear enough to give satisfactory results, and the level of the better ear is not of practical value without amplification. If one ear shows more limited frequency response or more recruitment than the other, it is best to use the hearing aid in the ear that responds more uniformly to all tones and that tolerates loud signals better.

If all the measurable aspects of hearing are the same in the two ears, the choice may be made on the grounds of convenience and appearance. The wearer may find it easier to insert the earpiece or to manipulate the cord and the case on one side than on the other. Planning for the use of the telephone or some listening device may indicate the preferred side. Even the cosmetic effect may be a determining factor.

The use of binaural receivers with a single hearing aid is so rare as almost to preclude consideration at the present time. Whatever theoretic advantages it might have are offset by practical and technical difficulties. However, there are instances in which it is advisable to have earpieces for both ears so that the hearing aid can be changed from side to side. Circumstances and personal judgments dictate the course to follow in this regard. We would seldom have a child switch his instrument from side to side without reviewing all the principles of advantage in each ear.

Final Selection—A Compromise

It is desirable, but unlikely, that all of these "best possible" features will be found in one instrument and in one ear. It is further desirable, and still more unlikely, that they will be achieved by the smallest, most durable, most inexpensive and best-serviced instrument available. Obviously then, we are faced with a series of compromises. Most people are willing to sacrifice a degree of quality and even of intelligibility for the sake of appearance and convenience. Some will inconvenience themselves by carrying larger instruments in order to hear better or to economize. None should sacrifice adequacy of performance for his particular needs for the sake of other advantages. It is appropriate that the audiologist or his equivalent preside and participate in many of the same compromises in selecting hearing aids for children that adults employ in making their decisions on an aid.

Davis states that "selecting a suitable hearing aid is, first, a series of tests of adequacy in fundamentals, and then a series of judgments of intangibles or a series of compromises. There is usually no one best fit that is demonstrably best under all circumstances." [3]

Older children usually can participate in enough of the tests of performance and judgments of comfort and quality to permit reasonably effective application of the foregoing principles. Even with younger children the improved instruments and techniques of observation along with prolonged study of behavior may reveal enough of their capacities to allow attainment of adequacy in the fundamentals of selecting hearing aids.

Acceptance of a Hearing Aid

Perhaps the most important aspect of placing a hearing aid on a child is that of making sure the instrument is accepted at least willingly at first and eagerly after a period of time. Attainment of this goal frequently requires a coordinated effort on the part of all those intimately associated with the child. The parents in particular must be willing and able to demonstrate acceptance of both the handicap and the means of alleviating it. If parents show feelings of anxiety and discontent over the child's condition, it will inevitably increase his sense of inadequacy.

ATTITUDE OF PARENTS

Actual emotional adjustment to their child's handicap may be utterly impossible for one or both parents for a period of time that would prove injurious to the child's progress. But even in the absence of desirable emotional reactions, it is not unreasonable to expect intelligent parents to act in such a way as to help the child feel comfortable in the new venture. If the parents can behave as though they accepted the hearing loss and the hearing aid objectively, and can maintain respect and love for the child in the face of these problems, it not only helps the child face his difficulties, but also helps the parents in their own deeper adjustments. This point bears emphasis since it is unrealistic to expect all parents to have developed before counseling or to acquire promptly after counseling the proper emotional attitude toward a handicapped child. Valuable as good counseling can be, it must not be expected that people can immediately start feeling as they should. However, it may be that they can learn in a short time to behave more appropriately as they gain insight into the problem. The proper behavior may then gradually produce results that bring about actual feelings of assurance and poise. For some parents emotional adjustment to a problem such as a hearing loss comes naturally and easily. For others, it takes a period of time and requires guidance. Unfortunately, certain parents may never be able to overcome their own feelings of guilt and inadequacy sufficiently to accept their child's handicap in a wholesome way.

Counseling of parents has proved to be helpful both in bringing about acceptance of a hearing problem and in pointing the way to a solution of the problem. Much individual counseling is done by physicians, teachers and others familiar with the problems of deafness. Physicians especially are in a position to give the kind of advice and encouragement that is needed. Accordingly, they face the serious responsibility of interpreting the problems of deafness realistically and at the same time hopefully. Physicians who are not properly equipped to examine and measure the function of the ears should be prepared to refer acoustically handicapped patients to qualified specialists or to appropriate clinics for further evaluation, treatment and guidance. Audiologists, of course, should be uniquely qualified to evaluate and interpret the communicative problems presented by a hearing impairment. They should know how to detect and to alleviate the grief and bewilderment that may prevail when parents are informed that their child has permanent loss of hearing. Teachers of the deaf and hard of hearing often can be of tremendous help in allaying anxiety and fear over the education and development of a child with a hearing loss. A visit to a school or clinic for the acoustically handicapped is usually a beneficial experience for parents. Other parents of similarly handicapped children and emotionally mature adults with hearing losses can give comfort and wise counsel to those who need assistance in facing the problems of deafness. Through one or more of these sources should come the assurance that deafness need not interfere with adequate growth and development of a child nor with his happiness and usefulness as an adult.

One of the most suitable and practical ways of counseling parents of acoustically handicapped children is to bring them together in small groups. Orientation sessions for parents of preschool children are conducted by a number of schools and clinics for the deaf and hard of hearing. Information on such programs from year to year may be found in each January issue of the American Annals of the Deaf, or may be obtained by writing to the editor of that journal.

Group meetings not only permit economic expenditure of time and effort on the part of teachers and counselors, but also provide effective emotional therapy. In addition to attending lectures, demonstrations and discussions on the function of hearing and the means of compensating for its loss, these parents have an opportunity to share and compare experiences and feelings with one another. This sharing of experience, plus a better understanding of the problem and the means of resolving it, may bring about the confidence and composure that are so important to the child's welfare.

In the instructional sessions the parents should be informed as fully as possible on the structure and function of the ear and the nature of hearing. The means of measuring hearing and the significance of the audiogram should be made clear. The parents should learn how and why reduced hearing affects the development of speech and language. Demonstrations of the acoustic effects of different types and degrees of hearing loss help the laymen to grasp these points. Each parent should be shown and made to understand the particular features of his child's hearing condition. Each should be told and shown what can be done by amplification. Information on the function, selection and use of hearing aids should be supplied. Finally, the principles and methods of training children with impaired hearing should be explained, demonstrated and practiced.

Attitude of Teachers and Playmates

While the attitude of parents is the most important factor in a child's adjustment to a hearing aid, it is well to give some attention to the way teachers and playmates react to the matter. Of course, teachers who have been trained to work with handicapped children know how to deal with the problems that arise from wearing a hearing aid. Regular classroom teachers, however, may feel inadequate when first faced with handling a child who wears a hearing aid. With the proper approach, it should not be difficult to prepare these teachers to treat the child naturally, and to accept the hearing aid just as they would glasses or a prosthesis of any kind. If a teacher understands the basic principles of a hearing aid and knows what hearing performance to expect of a particular child with an aid, she can arrange communication for him accordingly. After a teacher becomes comfortable in dealing with a hard of hearing child she can do a great deal to put the other children at ease with him.

If the proper example is set by adults, so that no embarrassment is evident, children are likely to show merely wholesome curiosity over a hearing aid. When circumstances permit, it is wise to explain to them the performance of a hearing aid and allow them to try it out. In this way their curiosity is satisfied, and very soon they are able to take the instrument for granted. If the wearer of the aid measures up in other respects, he too will be accepted by the group.

Learning to Wear a Hearing Aid

Along with the psychologic difficulties of accepting a hearing aid there is the very real physical burden to contend with. For small children a bulky instrument constitutes a serious incumbrance. Even smaller instruments on larger children are inconvenient. Every effort should be made to reduce the inconvenience as much as possible. For this reason it is desirable to select for a child as small and light an instrument as obtainable within the range of power and fidelity that is needed.

The arrangement for carrying the hearing aid should be given thoughtful attention. Either a special garment or appropriate pockets in certain types of clothing provide for stable placement of the instrument case. There should be no dangling of the instrument, and the friction between the case and clothing should be minimal. The use of a small holder made of flannel or other soft cloth into which the instrument fits tightly serves to reduce friction against the metal case and helps to hold it firmly in place. The instrument must be worn so that the microphone is not too close to the receiver. The distance between microphone and receiver necessary to eliminate feedback depends on the volume that is used and on the fit of the earpiece. The higher the volume used, the greater must be the separation of microphone and receiver. It is usually advisable to wear the microphone on the opposite side of the body from where the receiver is worn. If the earpiece does not fit properly in the ear or at the receiver coupling it may not be possible to separate the two units sufficiently to permit adequate volume. Difficulty along this line may necessitate a new earpiece from time to time.

CARE OF THE EARPIECE

In addition to fitting tightly enough for a good acoustic seal, the earpiece must be entirely comfortable. The child should be taught very early how to insert it properly and how to remove it without discomfort to the ear. The earpiece should be cleaned regularly. It may be washed with soap and water or rinsed in a special solution that is provided by some hearing aid dealers. Pipe cleaners are suitable and handy for removing wax that tends to accumulate in the canal of an earpiece.

CARE OF THE CORD

The care and manipulation of the receiver cord, like that of the earpiece, is as important as it is simple. The child should learn to arrange the cord over his ear and down the side of his neck in such a way that it does not gap nor become entangled in the clothing. Most wearers like the cord to lie under the shirt or dress collar, and to extend under the outer clothing to the place where the amplifier is worn. Small safety pins or eyelets in the clothing to anchor the cord at various points help keep it from working out of place or pulling uncomfortably on the wearer. Care in selecting a cord of the right length also makes for convenience and comfort as well as longer cord life. A spare cord should be kept on hand or be available on short notice. Either a child or an adult can easily learn to check the operation of a receiver cord and to change cords if one is faulty.

CARE OF BATTERIES

A young child will need assistance in the maintenance of batteries for his hearing aid. However, he will learn how very early and want to change the batteries himself. By matching the plus and minus signs on the batteries with those in the battery compartments of the instrument he will be able to insert new batteries properly. A child can and should learn that batteries are being drained when the instrument is turned on and are at rest when it is turned off. With this fact established, the habit should be fixed firmly of always turning off the instrument when it is not in use. Mastery of this one basic rule will do much to alleviate one of the worst problems encountered with hearing aids. It can be readily understood also that the battery compartments and the contact points must be kept clean. Since depleted batteries are likely to swell and leak corrosive fluid, one of the chief precautions in caring for the instrument is to make sure that worn-out batteries are not left in the case. It is often recommended that the "A" battery of vacuum tube instruments be removed each night.

As the child matures and learns numeric values he will want to know how to test and evaluate the voltage of his batteries. He will become interested in knowing and following the techniques of getting maximal service from the batteries. At this stage he may learn to use a voltmeter and to know at what levels the batteries become inadequate for proper operation. The principle of battery recuperation and the practice of rotating the use of certain types of batteries may be understood. Other battery principles such as recharging with an electric current, or depolarizing by air, may be encountered. In view of the constant developments and presently rapid changes occurring in hearing aids, particularly in regard to battery supply and maintenance, it is imperative that whoever directs a child's use of a hearing aid be informed on the management of the particular instrument that is used. Responsible and competent hearing aid representatives can be of great help in teaching the necessary facts and skills for operating their instruments efficiently and economically.

As early as possible a child with a hearing aid should be given full responsibility for the operation and care of his instrument. When he is able to take it off and put it on at will, to check and change the batteries and cords as needed, and to keep the entire instrument cleaned and polished, he will experience a sense of pride and independence.

SUCCESS WITH A HEARING AID

After the initial anxiety over putting on a hearing aid has subsided, the sustained attitude of the wearer will depend to a large measure on the degree of satisfaction gained from it. For this reason, it is of utmost importance that the early experiences a child has with his hearing aid be successful and as pleasurable as possible. Success with a hearing aid can be achieved by regulating the type and difficulty of the listening situation in which it is used. For instance, a child in the early stages of adjusting to an aid might not be expected to experience success or pleasure from playing a game in which there is a "cross fire" of conversation, but he may understand and enjoy a story told clearly in a quiet environment. The amount of regulation necessary and the type of situation suitable for early auditory experience depend, of course, on the efficiency of hearing attained with the hearing aid and on the child's speech and language comprehension. It is apparent that skill and practice of speech reading coupled with use of a hearing aid will improve understanding and thus enhance the interest and success in both skills. Further discussion of the principles and practices of auditory training and of speech reading may be found in other chapters of this book. In this regard I would only emphasize that the learning of speech reading is facilitated by the use of a hearing aid, and that the interpretation of what is heard is improved by the practice of speech reading.

References

1. GOLDSTEIN, M. A.: The Acoustic Method for the Training of the Deaf and Hard-of-hearing Child. St. Louis, The Laryngoscope Press, 1939, p. 26.
2. DIX, M. R. AND HALLPIKE, C. S.: The peep show: A new technique for pure tone audiometry in young children. Brit. Med. J. 2:719–723, 1947.
3. DAVIS, HALLOWELL: Hearing and Deafness: A Guide for Laymen. New York, Murray Hill Books, 1947, p. 206.

Bibliography

DAVIS, HALLOWELL: Hearing and Deafness: A Guide for Laymen. New York, Murray Hill Books, 1947.
HIRSCH, I. J.: The Measurement of Hearing. New York, McGraw-Hill, 1952.

MANDL, MATTHEW: Hearing Aids: Their Use, Care and Repair. New York, Macmillan, 1953.

SALTZMAN, MAURICE: Clinical Audiology. New York, Grune & Stratton, 1949.

WATSON, L. A. AND TOLAN, THOMAS: Hearing Tests and Hearing Instruments. Baltimore, Williams & Wilkins, 1949.

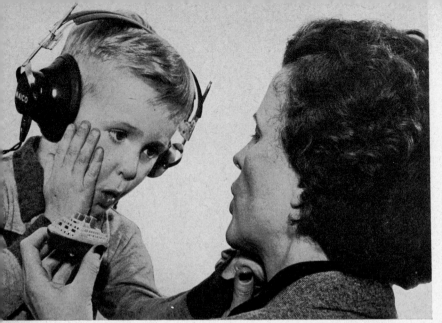

6

General Educational Aspects
of Hearing Loss

THE previous chapters have described how loss of hearing leaves its impact on the total development of the child. The educator views as his major concern the establishment and maintenance of a mode of communication with all acoustically handicapped children through which their social, intellectual, emotional and spiritual growth may be fostered. When a child is shut off from auditory stimuli the process of learning to communicate orally fails to develop. Even if a child is deprived of only a portion of his hearing he may find considerable difficulty in learning speech and language.

There is a basic disagreement among educators of children with profound hearing losses as to the best mode of communication for them. There are those who assert that many of these children cannot learn to understand the spoken word or to speak intelligibly. They recommend that these children be taught to read and write fluently but that the sign language * and the manual alphabet be substituted for oral communication.

Those who oppose this point of view contend that these children *can* learn to understand spoken language and *can* gain sufficient facility in expressing themselves orally to justify the time, effort and infinite diligence required to establish oral communication.

The two points of view as outlined here are an oversimplification of a very complex problem which originated in Europe with the rise of organized education of the deaf in the 18th and 19th centuries, and which has been passed down to the present. Arguments can be marshalled on both sides of the question, arguments which may sound convincing and logical, however emotional, depending on one's point of view. The truth of the matter still lies hidden in the future, for only further basic research can clarify the problem and resolve the controversy.

The assumption upon which this chapter and the following two are based is that children with impaired hearing are able to learn to communicate orally. Their education will be discussed from this point of view.

American education has long been committed to the principle that handicapped children are entitled to an education which meets their needs. The needs of the acoustically handicapped children vary widely because the group is not a homogeneous one. In it are some children who have been handicapped from the time of birth or shortly thereafter, and others who have lost their hearing later in life. The problems of the latter, the deafened children, differ from those whose losses stem from infancy,

---

* In the sign language a system of conventionalized gestures conveys units of thought without the use of words, or without regard to order of spoken language. The manual alphabet uses finger representations of the alphabet to spell out words to form sentences in their correct order.

for by the time they have lost their hearing they have already learned to communicate orally. They must, however, learn new ways of perceiving speech through the eye, rather than through the ear. They frequently require sympathetic guidance during the difficult period which follows deprivation of hearing. Among the children who have been handicapped from birth are those who can learn language and speech by ear alone; those who have considerable difficulty in understanding language by ear alone; and those who cannot learn it at all through the ear.

The terms "the deaf," "the hard of hearing" and the "deafened" are not intended to be descriptive of the diverse abilities of these children, so it is essential for purposes of discussion of their educational needs to arrive at a classification which delineates their characteristics in relation to language and speech development. The following classification refers to the children whose losses are irremediable and who have had impaired hearing from a time before which language was established.

CLASS 1. They are the children with *mild* losses (20–30 db in the better ear in the speech range). They learn speech by ear and are on the borderline between the normally hearing and those with significant defective hearing.

CLASS 2. They are the children with *marginal* losses (30–40 db). They have difficulty in understanding speech by ear at a distance of more than a few feet and in following group conversation.

CLASS 3. They are the children with *moderate* losses (40–60 db). They have enough hearing to learn language and speech through the ear when sound is amplified for them and when the auditory sense is aided by the visual.

The children in these first three categories may be considered as being hard of hearing.

CLASS 4. They are the children with *severe* losses (60–75 db). They have trainable residual hearing but their language and speech will not develop spontaneously, so they must learn to communicate through the use of specialized techniques. They are on the borderline between the hard of hearing and the deaf, and may be considered the "educationally deaf" or partially deaf.

CLASS 5. They are the children with *profound* losses (greater than 75 db). They cannot learn to understand language by ear alone, even with amplification of sound.

In the perception of oral language the eyes of all acoustically handicapped children will be called on to supplement their ears, and the tactile sense of some to supplement their eyes and ears. Speech reading, auditory training and a trained tactile sense are the avenues through which these children will achieve perception. Special equipment and special classes or schools are among the resources available to help them to arrive at their goal of better communication.

SPEECH RECEPTION AS RELATED TO CHILDREN WITH IMPAIRED HEARING

Lip Reading

Children with normal hearing are constantly and lavishly bathed in a stream of spoken words. As a result of the myriad auditory impacts on their developing minds, a spoken language emerges. Their vision, however, is not excluded as an aid to understanding the speech of others. Children learn early to associate a particular person with a particular voice and to identify certain sounds as pleasant when accompanied by a smile, or threatening when accompanied by a frown. They usually turn their heads to face the speaker, especially in a noisy environment. But the auditory sense is the important one for them in the process of learning oral language.

On the other hand, children with hearing impairments depend on the eyes to supplement what hearing they possess. How much they depend on their eyes is in a large degree determined by the type and degree of their hearing loss. If they have little or no hearing, vision becomes the primary sense through which communication is established and maintained.

Lip reading or speech reading is an art which must be acquired by the person who receives his language stimuli through the visual sense. To appreciate what is involved in reading speech visually, it is only necessary to turn off the sound on a television receiver in the middle of an interesting monolog or a dialog. The uninitiated person may immediately become badly frustrated since he may perceive a great amount of gesticulating, bobbing of the head and other bodily movements. When he does happen to glance at the speaker's mouth he sees a jumble of rapid jaw and lip movements. If he perceives only a word here and there, he will surely have lost the thread of the discourse by this time. Perhaps he has difficulty in seeing the lip movements on the small screen, especially if shadows fall across the speaker's face. A good lip reader knows he must meet all of these hazards if he is to read lips. He makes general use of the speaker's gestures, expression and bodily changes to give him clues, but he must constantly give his closest attention to the speaker's articulatory movements. He unconsciously observes the accent, stress and rhythm of the sentence, for these aspects of speech also carry meaning. If his attention wavers for even a moment from watching the speaker's mouth, he misses what is said.

Lip reading has been likened to the transcribing of shorthand. The lip reader is required to derive meaning from the partial clues he observes as the articulators pass rapidly from sound to sound, some of which are invisible to him. The person who can piece together these fragments and instantaneously organize or synthesize them into meaningful wholes makes the best lip reader.

The stream of speech is made up of a series of consonants and vowels placed in well-coordinated syllables set in stressed and rhythmic patterns. They emerge as words, phrases and sentences which carry meaning. Under even the most favorable circumstances the visual aspects of speech are incomplete and ambiguous. Some of the consonant sounds such as *k, g,* and *ng* are not visible on the lips because they are produced within the mouth cavity. Others like *t, d,* and *n* are often obscure especially when combined in syllables and words with vowels such as *i* or *e* where the space between the teeth is narrow. Consonants such as *p, b,* and *m* and others which appear on each of the lines in column I of table 1, though visible may be confused with one an-

TABLE 1.—*Distribution of Sounds of Speech according to Visibility on the Lips*

	I Easily Seen on Lips			II Often Obscure			III Obscure		
Consonants	p	b	m	t	d	n	k	g	ng
	wh	w			l		h		
	f	v			r (unrounded)			y	
	sh ch	j							
	s	z							
	¹th	²th							
		r (rounded)							
Vowels	ou			ŭ			ē		
	oi			ah			ĭ		
	aw			ŏŏ			ā		
	er (rounded)			er (unrounded)			ĕ		
	ōō			ī					
	ă								
	ū								
	ō								

other since they appear identical on the lips. The listener hears *s* and *z,* for instance, as distinct and different sounds, but the lip reader sees them as one and the same movement. In like manner, words in which these homophenous sounds occur (sounds which look alike on the speaker's lips) may be mistaken for each other. Only in the context of the phrase or sentence can the words *time, type, dime* or *sat, sand, sad* be distinguished as carrying a particular meaning. Unless there is contrast in the visible shape of consonants and vowels as they follow one another in speech, meaning can be further obscured. For instance, in the phrase "work shirt," the consonants *w* and *sh* and the vowel *er* are visible since they are all revealed by a puckering of the lips. Because there is no contrasting movement between the first and second *er,* a sentence such as, "The man put on a work shirt," may remain meaningless to the lip reader until the thought is stated in another manner.

Since no two individuals speak in the same way, variations in the production of speech also contribute to the problems of the lip reader. People who neglect to move their lips or who tightly clamp their jaws while talking, and those who speak with pipes or cigars anchored firmly in their mouths are truly enemies of the lip reader. Extremely rapid, extremely slow or exaggerated speech is anathema to the lip reader also. It goes without saying that the speaker whom the lip reader appreciates is one who talks at a moderate rate with clearly articulated visible movements, facing the lip reader and finishing his sentences once he begins them.

Factors which seem to influence lip reading besides the clarity of delivery involve the content of the message and the responsiveness of the lip reader. Material within the range of a child's experience delivered in that language with which he is already familiar will be easy for him to read, while material which contains strange concepts, difficult vocabulary and abstract ideas will be impossible for him to decipher. Knowledge of the verb in a sentence tends to strengthen its meaning. Use of the passive voice tends to make the material more difficult, as does the inversion of the sentence order, clustering modifiers around the subject of the sentence and adding parenthetic expressions.

It is evident that the lip reader should have good eyesight. Correctable refractory defects should be taken care of before the child is expected to learn to read lips. There are great individual differences among lip readers which seem quite unrelated to age, intelligence, educational achievement and length of time of the training period. Pintner [1] reports a zero correlation between intelligence and lip reading ability. It is generally believed that little relationship exists between these two factors. Heider and Heider [2] report a correlation of 0.54 between educational achievement and ability to read lips. Utley [3] concludes that lip reading ability cannot be predicted from school achievement.

Heider and Heider investigated several aspects of lip reading in their experimental study conducted at Clarke School for the Deaf. They report that children of the same chronologic age vary greatly in ability to read lips, that the yearly progress in lip reading as indicated by the difference between average scores of consecutive age groups is small, and that the differences are not due to disparities in the length of the training period. In investigating the role of motor organization in lip reading they found a correlation between ability to follow a rhythm in dancing and ability to read lips. They found the correlation between the ability to recognize vowels and lip reading much higher than that between the ability to recognize consonants and lip reading. They found no correlation between lip reading of nonsense syllables and general lip reading ability. There are many implications for the teacher in these studies. Lip reading, despite its limitations, is an art to be greatly cherished by the acoustically handicapped. Some children may require more help than others in acquiring this ability, but persistent effort, guidance and encouragement plus well planned programs should bring help to all who need it.

Auditory Training

Ability to make fine auditory discriminations is evident early in the lives of children who hear. By the time they have begun to talk they have sorted out the sounds of their native tongue from many other sounds which they accidentally produce, and they concentrate on imitating them. When they have reached the age of three or four they have mastered most of these sounds. If English speaking adults attempt to learn a foreign language they will undoubtedly attack the new language from the standpoint of their firmly established sensory habits. The results may be less than successful for in most persons ability to imitate new and strange sounds and unusual inflection patterns diminishes with age. For this reason modern practice tends to introduce programs of foreign language study early in the elementary grades. Just so, it is important to train the auditory sense of children with defective hearing as early as possible in order to utilize the flexibility of the young, to establish good consistent listening habits and to insure the best possible use of what hearing remains.

Fortunately the advent of the electric hearing aid has made it possible to bring sounds to the ears of children who might never have heard them without this help (see Chapter 5). Whereas the children who are fitted with glasses for the first time need no training in how to see through them, the children with defective hearing must be taught to use their hearing aids. They must learn how to adjust their aids, what to expect from them under varying conditions, how to listen to amplified sounds and to discriminate and interpret the sounds they hear. It is assumed that auditory training will be undertaken with the use of amplified sound, except for the unusual case where no hearing aid is indicated.

Under ordinary life conditions a person is called upon to recognize, distinguish between and interpret sounds which fall into three main categories (1) gross sounds, (2) musical sounds and (3) speech sounds. Gross sounds include all of the common sounds of the home, the neighborhood, nature and those produced by animals. They are the characteristic noises in the environment. Children with defective hearing are called upon to learn hundreds of words which describe these sounds: whimper, cry, growl, rattle, clang, roar, echo, resound, thunder, etc. The vocabulary related to this category of sounds is very extensive and should be emphasized when this aspect of auditory training is undertaken.

Musical sounds are very prevalent in the American culture by virtue of the popularity of television, radio and disc recordings. Children with hearing defects can learn to appreciate music—if not its idiom, certainly its rhythm. Rhythm is an important aspect of speech as well as of music, so it should be included in the school program.

The fifteen or sixteen vowel and twenty-five consonant phonemes which have symbolic value in English must be distinguished from one another if meaning is to be derived from spoken language. If a person hears, "He found the messy toad" when he should hear, "He found the missing coat," his mental picture may not relate to the facts in the situation. Individuals are called upon to interpret speech under both favorable and unfavorable conditions. An environment in which noise is predominant inhibits speech understanding. Children with defective hearing must first be given practice in recognizing and interpreting speech in a favorable situation before they are called on to sort out speech sounds from noises and to interpret speech sounds under adverse circumstances.

It had been assumed in the past that how a child reacted to auditory training depended largely upon the type and degree of his hearing loss. However, it is not uncommon to find that children with similar audiograms differ considerably in their responses to sound stimuli, even after long periods of training. Hopkins and Hudgins [4] suggest that even though it is not possible to predict from the audiogram how much a child will profit from auditory training, all acoustically handicapped children seem to derive some benefit from it, and should have every opportunity to continue training throughout their school lives.

By and large one may expect that a child with a mild conductive loss will learn language through his ear, though he might have difficulty in understanding quiet speech at a considerable distance. He hears and appreciates music and sings much as other children do (see table 2). When a child has a loss of 30 or 35 db in the better ear he begins to experience difficulty in hearing speech clearly beyond ten or fifteen feet. He has difficulty too in following a group conversation. Many of these children profit from wearing a hearing aid. A child with a moderate loss and an inner ear involvement, in which his perception of high frequencies is considerably diminished, has increasing difficulty in understanding speech because he is unlikely to be able to hear the soft speech sounds as f and th or the high pitched sounds, s, z, sh and ch. He may confuse k and t or g and d. He may never have heard a whisper or the ticking of a clock. He can, however, appreciate music and enjoy it.

A child with a perceptive loss of from 60 to 75 db is at a very

I Degree of Loss	II Effect of Hearing Loss on Understanding of Language & Speech	III Educational Needs
MILD 20–30 db	May have difficulty in hearing faint speech at distance Will experience no appreciable inconvenience in school situations Will not have defective speech as result of hearing loss	Speech reading Hearing aid—possible for selected young children with losses approaching 30 db Attention to vocabulary development Favorable seating
MAR-GINAL 30–40 db	Can understand average conversational speech at distance of 3 feet Can carry on face to face conversation without difficulty May miss as much as 50% of class discussion if voices are faint or not in line of vision May exhibit slight speech anomolies if loss is of high frequency type May exhibit limited vocabulary	Speech reading Individual hearing aid if prescribed and training in its use Speech training if necessary Attention to vocabulary development Favorable seating and possible special class placement for primary or selected children
MOD-ERATE 40–60 db	Can understand loud conversation at about 3 feet Misunderstands unwittingly Will have increasing difficulty in school situations requiring participation in group discussions May have defective speech if loss is high frequency type: difficulty with s, z, sh, ch, j: substitution of t and d for k and g, etc. Will very likely be deficient in language usage Will have evidence of limited vocabulary	Speech reading Individual aid if prescribed and auditory training. Also training with group aid as hearing loss approaches 60 db Speech training Special help in language arts: vocabulary development, usage, reading, writing English, etc. Favorable seating and/or special class placement for more severely handicapped in elementary school
SEVERE 60–75 db	May be able to hear moderate voice at several inches from ear Will hear loud noises at some distance: auto horns, dogs barking Speech and language do not develop spontaneously. Voice has good quality May be able to discriminate between vowels but not all consonants at close range	Speech reading Individual aid if prescribed and auditory training on individual and group aids Integrated language development and speech program by special teachers Special class on elementary level except for selected students in regular elementary school. Regular classes for selected high school students
PRO-FOUND 75 db +	May hear loud shout one inch from ear to no response at all Unaware of loud noises but may respond reflexively to loud sounds close to ear Speech and language do not develop spontaneously	Speech reading Auditory training on group aid and on individual aid if prescribed Special techniques required to develop language and speech through visual, auditory and tactile stimuli Special class or school indicated for elementary children. Regular classes only for selected high school students

great disadvantage in learning speech and language. He may not even hear the louder gross sounds or the rattling of a door knob, the tinkle of the door-bell or the crumpling of paper. Even with strong amplification he will have difficulty in discriminating some of the consonant sounds, though he may be able to identify and recognize many of the vowel sounds. He may still have a pleasantly inflected voice, but his articulation is likely to be defective. He still can enjoy music, but his pleasure in it is derived largely from its rhythm.

A child with a profound loss who hears only one or two frequencies may be able to distinguish the noise of a fire siren from that of a clap of thunder if they are close by, and he may be able to follow a musical rhythm aided by his tactile sense. He will be unable to make any of the finer discriminations between sounds necessary for the understanding of speech. However, there is evidence that ears do aid the deaf child in speech perception. Hudgins [5] reports a study in which word lists were read to children under three conditions: (1) children looked at the speaker only, (2) children looked and listened with hearing aids turned up to optimum level, (3) children turned up hearing aids to optimum level but did not look at speaker. The scores obtained from the second test where hearing and vision were both used were significantly higher than in tests where either sight or hearing were used alone.

It is a well known fact that the use of hearing and sight together for the hard of hearing is the most helpful solution to their speech perception problems. The knowledge that deaf children, though they are unable to interpret speech by hearing, can profitably use even a tiny bit of hearing to advantage should make a significant contribution to educational practice.

The Tactile Sense

The tactile sense is utilized as a supplement to sight and hearing when either of these two senses, or both, are profoundly affected. Deaf-blind children who are taught orally are primarily dependent on the tactile sense for their speech perception. Helen Keller, famous deaf-blind woman, "listens" to a speaker by placing her hand on the mouth and adjoining portions of the speaker's face. Deaf-blind persons learn to communicate in this extraordinary fashion only through continual practice and individual instruction in the tactile interpretation of speech. Children with good vision but little hearing also get valuable clues concerning the pitch of the voice, duration or length of the various sounds of speech, and the rhythm of sentences by placing their hands on the sides of the speaker's face. Vibrating diaphragms, such as those produced by stretching paper tautly over the wide end of a megaphone, or electrically driven ones, have been devised to train the tactile sense. These have been superseded in modern educational programs. However, the tactile sense, used in conjunction with vision and hearing is for many children the answer to their speech perception problems. Children with hearing defects are not bestowed with any special sensory gifts. If their achievements seem remarkable, it is because they have learned to use their senses in an exceptional manner.

LANGUAGE AND ITS EXPRESSIVE ASPECTS AS RELATED TO CHILDREN WITH IMPAIRED HEARING

Language

Most children have accomplished man's most outstanding intellectual feat—the mastery of spoken language—by the time they are ready for kindergarten. They have passed so easily and gradually through successive stages of language understanding and speech development that little thought is generally directed to how this amazing phenomenon occurs.

During the first 10 months of life, children's vocalizations are largely random, but they react to words of others before they are a year old (table 3). By then, most of them can imitate and produce one or two words independently. In their second, third and fourth years their vocabularies grow at an amazing rate and they come to use phrases and sentences orally to express their thoughts and their emotions. All this is accomplished without conscious effort.

There are two aspects to learning language: (1) achieving facility in the use of words which make up the language and (2) gaining control of its grammar. Acquisition of vocabulary is a life-long process which is related largely to experiences and needs. Young children with their limited experiences need a comparatively small vocabulary, whereas adults find expanded vocabularies necessary to meet their environmental demands.

TABLE 3.—*Age in Months at which Selected Language Items are Reported in Eight Major Studies in Infant Development (after McCarthy)*

Vocalizes 1	Says 1 word 11–14
Coos and babbles 2	Adjusts to simple
Responds by turning head	commands 12
to voice 4	Says 2 words 12
Vocalizes in self-initiated	Uses expressive jargon ...15
vocal play 4	Says 5 words 15–18
Distinguishes between	Names 1 object 17
friendly and angry	Names 2 objects 18½
talking 6	Joins 2 words in speech ..20
Vocalizes 2 syllables, as	Says first pronoun, phrase
da-da 7	and sentence 23
Utters single consonant ..8	Understands 2
Listens to familiar words ..8½	prepositions 25
Imitates sounds 9	Names 5 pictures 30
Imitates words 11½	

At the same time that sheer numbers of words are being added to those that an individual already knows, he must gradually become aware of the multiple meanings of words to express countless numbers of ideas. If a child is familiar only with the concepts related to "grow" and "little" in the sentence: "The little tree grew tall and strong," he will be completely unable to comprehend the meaning of a statement such as "The tadpole's tail grew shorter little by little."

Young children with mild hearing losses may show a little retardation in vocabulary development, while the ones with marginal losses which approach 35 db in the better ear will show a definite tendency toward having a limited vocabulary unless special effort is made to help relate verbal symbols to their experiences. The trend continues in intensified fashion with children in each of the succeeding classes mentioned above. For little deaf children the world of words does not even exist. They must learn that there is such a thing as language. They must learn that words are symbols which represent objects or ideas, and that these words can be arranged in a variety of sequences to express thoughts.

Modern English depends a great deal on arrangements of its constituent elements to carry meaning. Earlier forms of English depended on flexional endings of verbs, nouns, adjectives and articles to do this. As a consequence it did not matter whether a particular word stood first, second or third in the sentence. Its form told whether it was an object, subject or verb. Present-day English has largely discarded these word endings. Only the nominative and possessive forms of its nouns have been retained. Its articles and adjectives are not declined at all. "Content" words such as *coat, chair, doll, run, catch,* and *try* cannot today be easily identified as belonging to one part of speech or another, except as they appear in structures which in themselves signal meaning. For instance, in the following two sentences the word "doll" appears first as a noun, second as an adjective and then as a verb.

"Put the *doll* in the *doll* buggy."

"She likes to *doll* up."

English has also developed a wide use of words which have no other meaning than a grammatical or functional one. In the sentence "Do you see that bird at the top of the tree?" the words *do, at* and *of,* along with many other such words, are used to show relationships of the content words to each other and in themselves signal meaning only in the structures in which they appear.

Although modern English-speaking children are not burdened with learning numerous forms for every word in their vocabularies, they must acquire automatic control over very complex but basic word-order patterns. Children who hear do this even though they are confronted by a heterogeneous mixture of these patterns, and though no effort is made to present consistent repetitions of them.

Children with mild or marginal hearing losses will, no doubt, learn to use English naturally if their environments are conducive to it. Their language will be idiomatic and colloquial. Children with moderate losses will likely make language errors as a consequence of their deficient hearing. If such a child says: "My father work in the garden," it may be because he has not heard the "s" or the "ed" ending of the verb "work" as it was spoken in his presence. Errors of agreement between subject and verb, and in verb tenses may be quite common. It is difficult to isolate the problems of this group as being either speech problems or language problems. Whatever they are, it is necessary to integrate the learning of the structure of language with the speech needs of these children in the framework of their experiences.

"Educationally-deaf" children and deaf children have to be taught all the fundamentals of sentence structure. Only a systematic approach and carefully executed plan of language teaching will assure these children of a satisfactory facility with the use of language. At best, the language of deaf children who have attended school for several years is less mature than that of hearing children. Their teachers must be thoroughly grounded in the intricacies of English if they are to help them formulate clear concepts of our language. They must use every significant experience of the children to establish these concepts and lose no opportunity to guide the children in applying their knowledge in meaningful situations.

Writing or printing is merely a way of recording a language. Neither one is the language itself, since language is fundamentally an oral process. Hearing children are expected to learn to read and write only when they are ready to do so, readiness depending on mental age, experience and control over oral language. Only then are printed symbols substituted for familiar oral symbols. It seems reasonable that if oral communication is the aim for acoustically handicapped children the oral form of language must precede the written or printed form. Hard of hearing children who learn oral language naturally, learn to interpret printed symbols and learn to read at ages comparable to their brothers and sisters, though more attention must be devoted to the development of their vocabularies and to clarifying unfamiliar verbal concepts.

For deaf children the situation is a bit more complicated. If we waited until a deaf child had a vocabulary and language ability commensurate with that of a hearing first-grader, he might be ten or twelve years old before he saw a printed word. As soon as a deaf child has a good understanding of the nature of oral communication he is introduced to the printed symbols. This does not mean that oral presentation has not preceded the written; the lapse of time between the oral and written presentation may be very short. The printed symbol helps the deaf child to comprehend sentence structure more quickly and easily than without this aid, since his visual perception of it may be incomplete or even incorrect.

Speech

Speech is sometimes referred to as an overlaid function, since all the organs of speech have basic vegetative functions. Breathing supplies the body with oxygen but also serves as the motor power of speech. The closure of the glottis (space between the two vocal chords) protects the air tract during the act of swallowing, and in fixation of the thorax provides extra power for acts requiring firm forceful action by the upper part of the body. This is the point at which voice is initiated. The mouth, nose and throat serve as passageways for food and air to their respective destinations, but also act as resonators in speech production. By changing the size and shape of those cavities, resonant frequencies are changed, thereby influencing the quality of the sounds produced. The tongue, lips and palate have important basic functions in chewing and swallowing, but are also the main organs of articulation. All of the activities associated with speech: breathing, vocalizing and articulating are closely coordinated in the production of spoken language.

Children with defective hearing have this necessary anatomic equipment to produce speech. Some will learn to use the speech mechanism naturally, while others will have to be taught to do so. Those with mild or marginal losses will generally have no speech defects. If they do, it is not likely that the hearing loss is responsible. Those whose hearing is diminished considerably, and who have inner ear impairments, may have difficulty in producing sounds of speech such as *s, sh, ch, t* or *k,* which they do not hear clearly even with amplification. Their problem is to learn to perceive these sounds through visual stimuli and to rely on the kinesthetic or muscle sense to incorporate them into their speech. These children generally have good voices. Every effort has to be made, however, to insure retention of good voice quality and to preserve what good articulation the children have.

Those who have losses as great as 60 db, even though they do not learn language spontaneously, have the great advantage of having trainable residual hearing to aid them in speech perception and production. These children too must depend upon the kinesthetic sense to guide them in the production of sounds they do not hear. Deaf children, those with profound losses, cannot produce speech except after being taught by artificial rather than by natural means. Though they babble much as hearing children do in infancy they do not retain what sounds they produce, since they have no auditory sense to reinforce their vocalizations. Deaf children have to learn to vocalize on a conscious level. They have to learn to control the pitch of their voices and to make the fine adjustments of the articulators, guided almost entirely by their kinesthetic senses; and they must coordinate all of these movements with breathing. It is no wonder then that the speech of deaf children tends to be less intelligible than is desirable. Hudgins and Numbers [6] attribute the failure of deaf children generally to achieve intelligibility to a lack of integration and coordination of the many muscle groups which are used in the production of speech. The teaching of speech must be integrated with learning of language if oral communication is to be achieved by deaf children.

ORGANIZATION OF EDUCATIONAL SERVICES FOR
CHILDREN WITH HEARING IMPAIRMENTS

The education of children with impaired hearing should be basically the same as that which is desirable for all American children who are to grow up into responsible citizens in a democracy. Though the special educational needs of these children center around the development of communication skills, many factors enter into the determination of how and where they will receive their education. These factors include, besides those just discussed, their age, intelligence, physical status, social maturity and the availability of services.

In a metropolitan area which is cognizant of the needs of its handicapped children there will be many types of services for children who have hearing difficulties. Those whose language and speech are commensurate with those of children in their own age groups will be able to attend regular elementary or high schools and receive the special help they need from teachers who are specially trained in speech perception techniques, speech therapy and principles of language development. These children will be visited once or twice weekly by itinerant teachers, or they will go to centers where a teacher has her headquarters. Included in this group will be practically all of the children with mild or marginal hearing losses, most of those with moderate losses, a small number with severe losses and very few deaf children. Children with severe and profound losses who have to compete with their peers in such a situation must be well adjusted, must have good minds and a strong drive to succeed. They cannot be the kind who are easily frustrated, for they will encounter many difficulties during the course of their school lives.

For children whose language and speech is only partially developed or is quite deficient, placement in special classes for the acoustically handicapped will be indicated. They need intensive daily help in developing speech and language, and can best receive it under the direction of specially trained teachers. This group may include children with moderate, severe and profound losses. Opportunity for association with hearing children may be on a nonacademic level, as in kindergarten activity or play periods or in art and gym classes. In certain selected situations where the regular classroom teacher is a sympathetic, understanding person, and where the stresses and strains are not too great for the handicapped, the children may jointly participate in arithmetic, spelling or other academic classes. The emotionally immature, the slower learners or the poorer lip readers often find the security of the special classes preferable to participation in regular classroom activities.

In large communities there may be a special day school for deaf children. It may be housed in conjunction with an elementary school or it may be an institution set off by itself. At the present time about 27 per cent of all children enrolled in schools for the deaf attend special day classes or schools. Most are students in the public residential schools scattered throughout the United States.[7]

If a child lives in a rural community or in a small village which maintains no services for handicapped children, he may not be able to receive his education at home. Children with mild or marginal losses may be able to adjust to the regular program if they are under the guidance of intelligent teachers who are aware of the children's problems. In some consolidated school districts it has been found expedient for several communities to share a teacher who has been trained to help children with mild or moderate impairments. Children with greater losses may experience enough difficulty, even with considerable help, to warrant placement in special classes away from home.

If, in addition, the child has another disability such as low intelligence, reduced vision or cerebral palsy he will have to be placed in a situation which deals mainly with his primary handicap. Provision must be made for his secondary handicap within the framework of the first. Many hard of hearing children will be found in schools of the orthopedically handicapped, and mildly cerebral palsied children will be found in classes for deaf children. Mentally retarded hard of hearing children may find their needs best satisfied in classes for the mentally retarded, while mentally retarded deaf children may need special placement within the organization of the classes for the acoustically handicapped. No hard and fast rules can be laid down for the education of any individual child. The prime objective is to make adequate provision for the changing needs of each as he grows and develops. Only when a child's needs and capabilities have been carefully evaluated and periodically re-evaluated can his placement be determined.

REFERENCES

1. PINTNER, R.: Speech and speech reading tests for the deaf. Am. Ann. Deaf 74:480–486, 1929.
2. HEIDER, F. AND HEIDER, G.: An Experimental Investigation of Lip-Reading. In Studies in the Psychology of the Deaf. Psychol. Monogr. No. 1, 1940.
3. UTLEY, JEAN: Factors involved in teaching and testing lip-reading ability through the use of motion pictures. Volta Review 48:657–659, 1946.
4. HOPKINS, LOUISE AND HUDGINS, C. V.: The relationship between degree of deafness and response to acoustic training. Volta Review, 55:32–35, 1953.
5. HUDGINS, C. V.: Problems of speech comprehension in children. Nerv. Child 9:57–63, January 1951.
6. HUDGINS, C. V. AND NUMBERS, FRED: An investigation of the intelligibility of the speech of the deaf. Genet. Psychol. Monogr. 25:289–392, 1942.
7. American Annals of the Deaf, January 1954.

BIBLIOGRAPHY

American Annals of the Deaf, January issue.
BEST, HARRY: Deafness and the Deaf in the United States. New York, Macmillan, 1941, chaps. XXII–XXIII.
BLOOMFIELD, LEONARD: Language. New York, Henry Holt, 1933.
DELAND, FRED: The Story of Lipreading. Washington, D. C., The Volta Bureau, 1931, chaps. I–IX.
FRIES, CHARLES C.: The Structure of English. New York, Harcourt Brace, 1952. ———: Teaching and Learning English as a Foreign Language. Ann Arbor, University of Michigan Press, 1945.
HEIDER, F. AND HEIDER, GRACE: A Comparison of Sentence Structure of Deaf and Hearing Children. In Studies in the Psychology of the Deaf. Psychol. Monogr. No. 1, 1940.

HUDGINS, CLARENCE V.: Problems of speech comprehension in children. Nerv. Child 9:57–63, January 1951.

—— AND HOPKINS, LOUISE: The relationship between degree of deafness and response to acoustic training. Volta Review 55:32–35, January 1953.

McCARTHY, DOROTHEA: Language Development in Children. In Handbook of Child Psychology (Carmichael, ed.). New York, John Wiley & Sons, 1946.

PEI, MARIO: The Story of Language. Philadelphia, J. B. Lippincott, 1949.

PINTNER, RUDOLPH: Speech and speech reading tests for the deaf. Am. Ann. Deaf 74:480–486, 1929.

UTLEY, JEAN: Factors involved in teaching and testing lip-reading ability through the use of motion pictures. Volta Review 48:657–659, 1946.

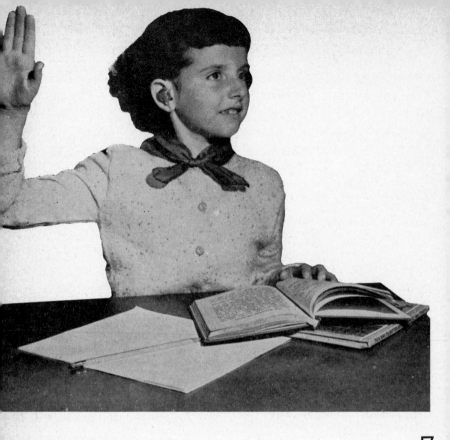

7

Education of Children with Mild and Moderate Hearing Losses

THE PRESCHOOL CHILD

The Role of the Parents

THE child's first and most important teachers are his parents, and one of their most significant functions is the guidance of his emotional development. They have it in their power to mold him into a happy well-adjusted child, or into a belligerent, withdrawn or unhappy individual. Good adjustment within the family is just as basic to the child's school progress as his in-

184

telligence or degree of hearing loss. The child who comes to school emotionally secure is free to learn, and may be expected to direct his energy toward whatever educational goals are set up for him, while one who is deeply disturbed and continually upset cannot be expected to attack his school problems successfully.

Parents who have good mental health themselves and constructive attitudes toward their child's hearing loss will be able to do most in preparing the young hard of hearing child for school. Such parents will seek out ways in which to help the child fit happily into the family situation, not by coddling him, excusing him or covering up for him, but by acknowledging the existence of his hearing loss and making the necessary adjustments to it.

Mr. and Mrs. Revere were just such parents. On the advice of their doctor they enrolled in a class for parents of children with impaired hearing shortly after they had discovered through a well-baby clinic that their two-year-old son, Ricky, had a hearing loss. They realized that their part in Ricky's early training was vital. This class was conducted under the auspices of an audiologic clinic which was an adjunct to a large university hospital in their community. Here they attended a weekly series of ten evening meetings where they listened to lectures by doctors, audiologists, psychologists and educators, participated in discussions, saw movies and watched demonstrations of lip reading and auditory training.

They learned that all children followed certain patterns of physical, mental and social growth, that each child proceeded at his own individual rate and that children with hearing losses were no different in this respect from any other children. They became aware that learning was a spontaneous experience in young children and occurred largely by way of example rather than by admonition, exhortation or formal teaching. They also learned about how the ear is constructed and how it functions, what may interfere with its proper functioning, and what measures may be taken when medical means cannot restore it. They learned what an audiometer test was and had the experience of taking a test themselves. They found out about the different types of hearing aids—their virtues and limitations—and got advice about when to purchase an individual aid for their child. They discovered how to entice a child to wear earphones by

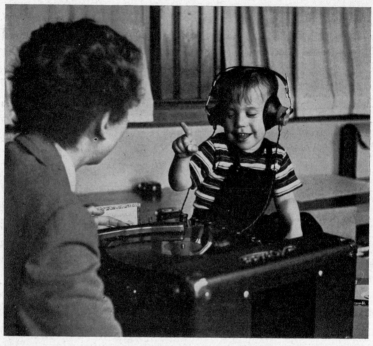

Ricky's parents, through observation at the audiologic clinic, learned to make listening meaningful as well as fun for him.

wearing them themselves while listening to television or to a record player. They found out the importance of having their child within easy seeing-hearing distance of them when they wanted to talk to him and not shouting to him when he was in another room, but either going to him or having him come to them when they called his name. They began to realize that it was important to talk to him a great deal, more so than if he did not have a hearing loss. They learned that when they talked to him they were to speak clearly and distinctly and in language that they would use if they were speaking to any other two-year-old. They were convinced too, that it was important to explain his handicap to their friends and relatives, and as Ricky grew older, to his playmates and their families. This they did, without being secretive about it or without calling undue attention to Ricky's hearing loss in his presence, for he *could* hear them when they talked about him.

By the time Ricky was ready for kindergarten his hearing aid was a familiar part of him. He had learned to look and listen when people spoke to him, so he learned language easily and naturally and spoke intelligibly and fluently. Ricky was a well adjusted, intelligent hard of hearing child whose parents started him off on the right path toward meeting his own special problems with equanimity.

Importance of Early Education

The early education of hard of hearing children is crucial, for it utilizes the child's great need and desire to learn language, which are most intense during the preschool years. If there are no organized services in a community for the guidance of parents, the task devolves largely upon the special teacher. This is done through individual contacts: visits to the home, invitations to visit special lessons and occasional conferences at school. Parents who have the aptitude for training their preschool children easily, happily and informally at home should be encouraged to do so. Under some circumstances this may not be possible where both parents are employed or where the child has no playmates near his home. If a child is in an unhappy home situation it may be more desirable to enroll him in a nursery school for hearing children, but under no circumstances in a school for the deaf. The hard of hearing child should receive his education in the regular school.

THE SCHOOL PROGRAM

The Role of the Regular Class Teacher

Since hard of hearing children as a group tend to have more, rather than fewer, adjustment problems than normally hearing children and since all parents are not able by any means to give their children the guidance which is most desirable for the young, the school must be prepared to furnish a favorable environment in which the child's problems may be worked out as satisfactorily as possible. The child's teachers play an important role in his school adjustment. Although there are countless numbers of sympathetic, understanding teachers in today's schools there are equally as many who are emotionally unfit to become involved with the special problems of exceptional children, or who simply do not care to become involved. Basically, lack of knowledge about these children is at the root of this difficulty, and it stems from an incompleteness in most undergraduate teacher training programs as well as from a lack of inservice training programs later. Many teachers are harassed by large classes and feel that besides not being prepared to deal with exceptional children they do not have the time to pay attention to individual needs, much as they would like. These are personnel and administrative problems yet to be solved.

Fortunate indeed is the hard of hearing child who finds himself in a room with an alert and sympathetic teacher. She is aware of the individual needs of the hard of hearing child and is willing to make the small but important adjustments within her classroom to help ease the school situation for him. First of all, the hard of hearing child in her room has the privilege of changing his seat so that he may always be within range of seeing and hearing her and also his classmates. She does not talk and give directions when she is writing on the blackboard. She and the other children try to face the light as well as the child when they speak because they know it is difficult to read the lips of a silhouette. If the child does not understand, he is free to ask what she is talking about. She does not repeat word for word what she has said but rephrases her sentence, thereby adding a possible clue to what is being discussed. She may sometimes ask the child to repeat her directions to the class to be sure he has understood them.

She cooperates well with the child's special teacher. Together they work out a plan to interpret hearing loss to the child's classmates. They demonstrate how a hearing aid works and let the other children satisfy their curiosity by listening to it. The children discover that they do not need to raise their voices when speaking, for the hearing aid makes their voices loud enough to be heard. She allows the other children to attend the lip reading sessions with the hard of hearing child as a special privilege, for she knows that much is to be gained by doing this. Here the children learn that it is easy to misunderstand speech when it is not clearly heard. Though "funny answers" sometimes make others laugh, the mistakes of the lip reader may be legitimate ones. The hard of hearing child learns to laugh at his own mistakes too, but more important, all learn tolerance for each other. She and the special teacher plan the program of help in language and speech within the framework of the activities going on in her room.

The hard of hearing child in her class is truly an integral part of the group. He knows he has certain privileges which the others do not have, but he does not take advantage of them since he respects his teacher and his classmates as they respect him. He takes part in the plays, belongs to the scouts, is a classroom monitor or is elected a reporter for the class newspaper. This teacher is doing much to help all hard of hearing children. By setting up a permissive, understanding atmosphere in her classroom for the hard of hearing children, her group absorbs her philosophy and in turn consciously or unconsciously passes on its knowledge and understanding to others.

The Role of the Special Teacher

Because teachers in regular classes are not equipped to handle the special problems related to the development and maintenance of communication skills, specially trained teachers must be provided to do this for the hard of hearing children. An individual who chooses to work with hearing handicapped children should have a warm personality, a sincerity of purpose and the ability to work as a member of a team which is responsible for the child's educational and social development. Since not all regular classroom teachers are informed about the problems of hard of hearing children, it frequently becomes the task of the special teacher to interpret their needs to the classroom teacher as well as to their classmates and parents. She must be ever willing to speak before community groups to explain the problems of children with defective hearing. She must be able to outline their needs to the administrators of the school system. In short, she must be wise, diplomatic, patient and tolerant.

Though she is a specialist, the person who works with hard of hearing children should be a teacher first. She should have a good knowledge of teaching techniques, and of the school curriculum, for her work will be effective only to the degree that she can relate her therapy to what is going on in the child's classroom. She herself must have good hearing and speech and should have no physical abnormality of mouth or lips which would interfere with speech reading. Besides, she must have a thorough knowledge of speech perception techniques, speech and language development in normal children, and of correction of faulty speech. She should be familiar with the construction of hearing aids, be able to operate them efficiently and detect inadequate performances of the aids. She should be able to interpret medical and psychologic reports and to administer audiometric tests and tests of educational achievement and social maturity.

This teacher may be a properly trained speech correctionist who handles many types of speech disorders in the course of her travels from school to school or from class to class. Or she may be a person trained specifically to teach acoustically handicapped children, and be in charge of a special class which serves children with varying degrees of hearing loss. The hard of hearing children assigned to the center in which her class is housed may come to her several times a week, or daily, if their needs are best met this way. It is her responsibility to determine each child's special program in cooperation with the child's regular teacher or teachers.

THE SPECIAL PROGRAM

Determining Needs of Children

A careful study of the school records should reveal a great deal of valuable information which the special teacher will need in order to plan efficiently. From the records she should learn the children's ages, medical and developmental histories, family background, potentialities for intellectual growth, school progress, educational achievement, social maturity and personality problems, and, for high school students, their vocational interests. If she works in one of a number of growing communities she will find audiologic reports for hard of hearing children among the records. They contain (1) the otologist's report, (2) the pure tone audiometric tests of air and bone conduction, (3) speech audiometric measurements of threshold, of ability to hear at comfortable levels of loudness and of tolerance for loud sounds, and (4) recommendations for a hearing aid. If she has had a predecessor she should also find speech evaluation records for all the children who have received help in speech. In passing, it should be noted that she is responsible for keeping the records up to date and for completing the files for her successors.

More than likely, not all of the aforementioned reports will be readily available for all of her children. The special teacher will then have to take the initiative in securing data from such qualified individuals as the school psychologist and school social worker, or from related agencies as the Adult Vocational Rehabilitation office for children over 16, or from an audiologic clinic in or near her community. If she has no access either to records or to resources for furnishing this information she will of necessity have to be her own caseworker, and gather such information as will allow her to proceed in an intelligent systematic fashion in planning her work.[1,2]

Even though there is a complete file on a child she will still want to explore informally the child's ability (1) to read lips, (2) to perceive speech in the classroom situation with and without a hearing aid, and (3) to produce acceptable speech. On the basis of this information she will not only plan what special services each child will require, but how much and how often he will need her help.

Grouping for Special Services

In general, the special teacher will find that if she can group her hard of hearing children on the basis of their common interests, her work will be more stimulating, effective and interesting than if she limits herself to individual tutoring.[3] The itinerant teacher in many instances may have to meet the hard of hearing child alone for lip reading and auditory training if there is only one in a school she visits. If it is possible, she should place him in a speech group with other children who have speech problems but who are not hard of hearing.

The special teacher may actually choose to have a recently deafened child come to see her alone on occasion. During the period of emotional upheaval which ordinarily follows deprivation of the use of an organ or sense, the child needs warm-hearted guidance and an opportunity to talk out some of his problems privately. She may feel that he needs a concentrated lip reading-auditory training program to speed his readjustment to a regular class situation. If he is an adolescent he may rebel at the suggestion of wearing a hearing aid, since he abhors the thought of being different from his classmates. Therefore the teacher may find it advantageous to have this child also meet with other hard of hearing children so that he may see how matter-of-factly they accept their losses and wear their hearing aids. His adjustment to his new condition may be greatly expedited through group therapy.

Other children, as the child with one good ear and one deaf ear, and the child's classmates may be invited to join the lone child from time to time. The special teacher should not expect the child with a unilateral loss to be a regular member of a group, since one good ear is almost as good as two for learning speech and language. He may have some difficulty in localizing sounds because two good ears are necessary for this purpose.

Adjustments in seating arrangements in his classroom should alleviate any minor inconvenience he might encounter there.

In metropolitan communities where children are brought to a center, the special teacher will be able to group children on interest levels quite effectively. Her groups, nevertheless, are bound to be heterogeneous from the standpoint of degree and type of hearing loss, as well as of ability to read lips naturally. The teacher must therefore learn to individualize instruction within the group, a technique difficult to learn but most effective when mastered.

The time spent in each contact with primary grade children will be shorter than that spent with older children. Those who require a greater number of services will need more of the teacher's attention. Children who adjust easily to wearing a hearing aid and are also good lip readers will need a lesser total number of contacts than the poor lip reader, the poorly adjusted children or those who need tutoring in vocabulary and reading. Table 1 outlines roughly how often a teacher may schedule a child for help, keeping in mind his level of maturity, his interests and the amount of service he requires.

TECHNIQUES

Introduction

If hard of hearing children are expected to use the combined senses of hearing and sight in the perception of speech, it follows that the lip reading and auditory training programs must be closely integrated. Though in every lesson children will be expected to interpret speech by ear alone or by eye alone, some opportunity should also be given to use vision and hearing together. Speech rehabilitation may or may not be directly linked with the subject matter of the speech perception lessons. The very nature of the typical speech task for the hard of hearing —learning new muscular habits for the production of some speech sounds—implies that the process will be slow and repetitive. In any case, lip reading, auditory training and speech training should be closely related to the children's interests, experi-

TABLE 1.—*Schedule for Special Lessons for Hard of Hearing Children of Various Ages & Interest Levels*

Level in School	Degree of Loss	Min. Per Lesson	Lessons Per Wk.	Lessons Per School Year	Special Areas of Instruction	Levels of Interest *
Primary	mild	15–20	1	1 semester and then occasionally thereafter	lip reading auditory training	animals bikes caring for pets conducting roadside stands dramatization dolls and cars fairy tales here and now stories make believe playing house, school rockets, space ships
	marginal	20	2	1 yr. for good lip readers and occasionally thereafter	lip rd., aud. tr. (no speech)	
	moderate	30	2–5	continuing	lip rd., aud. tr., speech, tutoring in langage	
Inter-mediate	mild	20	1	1 semester and occasionally thereafter	lip reading	adventure biography collecting cards, airplanes, cars, etc. fairy tales foreign lands funnies and comics jokes nature mechanics science scouting skating, swimming, team games space ships spectator sports travel westerns
	marginal	20	2	1 yr. for good lip readers and occasionally thereafter	lip rd., aud. tr. (no speech)	
	moderate	30–40	2–5	continuing	lip rd., aud. tr., speech, tutoring in language arts	

Junior High	mild	30–40 or 1 period	every 2 weeks	1 semester, then occasionally	lip reading	sensational adventure exploration health movies mysteries science active team games sports travel
	marginal	30–40 or 1 period	1	1 yr. for good lip readers	lip rd., aud. tr. (no speech)	
	moderate	30–40 or 1 period	2–3	continuing	lip rd., aud. tr., speech, tutoring in language	
High School	mild	45–50 1 period	every 2 weeks	1 semester then occasionally	lip reading	community youth activities dancing dates developing talents earning money homemaking hobbies stamp collecting model airplanes knitting, etc. mechanics music, jive reading current best sellers romance mysteries sports: tennis, swimming, golf spectator sports social behavior vocational plans
	moderate	45–50 1 period	2	1 yr. for good lip readers	lip rd., aud. tr. (no speech)	
	severe	1 period	2–3	continuing	lip rd., aud. tr., speech, tutoring in subjects	

* After *How Children Develop*, Columbus, Ohio, Ohio State University, 1946.

ences and classroom activities. If there is to be tutoring in language and reading, planning with the classroom teacher is mandatory so that there will be a direct relationship between the special lessons and what is being taught in the regular classroom. Though the integration of the special services is assumed, the approaches to lip reading, auditory training and speech training will be discussed separately.

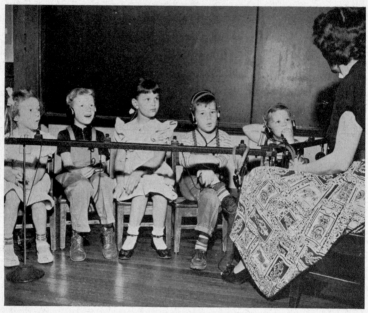

Two children wear individual hearing aids and the others use a group amplifier.

Lip Reading

The teacher of lip reading will have to rely largely on her own ingenuity and observation to discover a child's speech reading ability. The one standardized motion picture test of lip reading available requires a third grade level in reading.[4-5] It is a paper and pencil test, and about an hour is needed for its administration. The test is divided into three sections: the first, a set of 31 sentences or phrases; the second, a set of 36 single words; and the third, 6 episodes in each of which one or two speakers discuss an experience keyed to interests of children from the intermediate to the high school level. DiCarlo and Kataja,[6] who studied the test with a group of 99 adults composed of normally hearing and aurally handicapped individuals, concluded that it was longer than it need be, and was so difficult as to discourage even the most proficient lip readers. They suggested that the lack of situational clues contributed to its difficulty.

The teacher's first task is not to discourage her pupils, but to encourage them and to stimulate them to want to learn lip reading. She will want to use the first one or two contacts with the children to establish rapport with them and also to explore their abilities. This she can do by preparing interesting, not too difficult but yet challenging and appropriate material. Since there is a limited amount of published lip reading material suitable for use with children, she will have to prepare most, if not all of her own, if she is to take into account the interests and abilities of the children she teaches. A knowledge of the various approaches to teaching lip reading to adults as well as to children will be very helpful to her in preparing her lessons.

One of the earliest published books on lip reading for adults in the United States is that of Bruhn, whose translation from the German of the Mueller-Walle method was among the first real contributions to the literature in this country.[7] While acknowledging the need of synthetic power in the lip reader, Bruhn feels that the student must be aware of, and be able to analyze details. This, according to Bruhn, is to be accomplished through rapid rhythmic syllable drills. She introduces her lessons with a study of the positions assumed by the various articulators in the production of the elements of speech. In her first lesson (one of several basic lessons) she combines the more visible of the consonants, *p b m, s z, f v, sh ch, th* and *w wh* with vowels into open syllables as in *fō, fä*. By permutation of combinations of vowels and consonants she arrives at quite a complete series of syllable drills which are not to be interpreted as being meaningful speech. For instance, syllable drills presented in rhythmic patterns as:

$$sō\ fä\quad fä\ mē\quad mē\ shä$$
$$fä\ mā\quad sē\ fā\quad mā\ sō$$
$$mō\ sē\quad mä\ sē\quad mā\ sē$$

lead into paradigms as:

> They may . . . They may see . . .
> She may . . . She may see . . .
> We may . . . We may see . . .
> You may . . . You may see . . .

which in turn are expanded into sentences as:

> She may see the ship.
> You may see me sew.
> They may go to the farm.

Bruhn's lessons also include stories which are developed through phrase and sentence drills, as:

The bird flew away.
The bird flew away to a tree.
The bird flew away to a tall tree by the side of a river.
A cat saw the bird.
A wily cat saw the beautiful bird.
A wily cat saw the beautiful bird sitting on a tall tree by the side of a river.

After the entire story is prepared in this way the actual story is read and the students are questioned about it. A study of homophenes is also included in the lesson. In her revised text, Bruhn [8] suggests that written work be part of each lesson. Bruhn's book for children follows the same philosophy and pattern as that established in the text for adults.[9]

Another German method, the Jena Method, was introduced into the United States through the efforts of Jacob Reighard and Bessie Whittaker in 1927 and first published by Bunger [10] in 1932. This method was first devised by Karl Brauckmann as a means of teaching deaf children at the school for the deaf in Jena, Germany. It is based on the idea that of the five forms of speech as outlined in Bunger's book: the audible, the visual, the gestural, the mimetic and the movement form, the last is

the most important to the lip reader. It assumes that if the lip
reader can reproduce unconsciously the speech movements of
a speaker in his own speech musculature he will possess one of
the best means of interpreting what he cannot see or hear. The
paramount aim of this method is to develop kinesthetic awareness of speech. The lip reader first memorizes a basic vowel
series: ā, ē, ō, ah, aw, ĕ, ōō, ă, ū, ou, ī, oi, ŏŏ, ĭ, ŭ, er. These
vowels are then combined with consonants into syllables which
are presented in a variety of rhythmic patterns, as bā′ bē/ bō′
bah/ baw′ bĕ/ bōō′ bă/ bū′ bou/ bī′ boi/ bŏŏ′ bĭ/ bŭ′ ber/, and
reinforced with bodily movements such as clapping of hands
and bouncing of balls. The student speaks the chosen series of
syllables following the lead of the teacher who uses full voice
at first. Later, students follow when the teacher retires behind
a window so she cannot be heard. These syllables may or may
not lead to sentences:

lĕ lĕ lĕ lĕ   mē mē mē mē   caw caw caw caw   daw daw daw daw

> le′ me′ caw′ daw′
> le′ me′ caw′ daw′
> le′ me′ caw′ daw′
> Let me call the dog.

The sentence stress may be varied also. Sentences given in
the form of conjugations bridge the gap between the meaningless syllables and context materials.

The student is encouraged gradually to stop using his voice
and to follow the speaker with subvocal muscle movements.
When the teacher feels, after several weeks or months of syllable
drills, that her pupils have become kinesthetically aware of their
own and the speech of others, lessons built on subjects interesting to the students are begun. They include sentences and
stories. Current events, biographies, famous buildings, national
monuments and parks are among the topics suggested for the
college students to whom Bunger's book is directed.

The next method which merits attention is Nitchie's. He published his first text on lip reading in 1912, but his method as
it is known today was not crystallized until about 1919.[11] Be-

cause Nitchie believes that the teaching of lip reading is a psychologic problem, he stresses the importance of training the mind to grasp thoughts as a whole rather than the training of the visual memory for words or sounds. Therefore he suggests that each lesson begin with an anecdote—10 to 15 sentences long —read by the teacher and retold in his own words. The student interrupts for meaning after the first telling. The story is concluded when the student can answer questions about it. Conversational practice by student and teacher, which is based on such subjects as the restaurant, the doctor's call, or the weather, follows. The next portion of the lesson is devoted to a study of an articulatory "movement"; for instance, $\overline{oo}$ if it is a vowel, or f and v if it is a consonant. The "movement" $\overline{oo}$ would be observed as it appears in words such as *moon, soon* and *stoop*. Sentences based on the "movement" words are read and rephrased for meaning if the student does not understand the sentence after one repetition. For instance, if the sentence, "It will be time to go there *soon*," causes difficulty the teacher might say, "The movie will begin at seven o'clock. The movie will begin soon. It is almost seven o'clock. It will be time to go there soon."

Nitchie did not publish any books of materials suitable for children, but several based on his method have appeared in print.[12]

All other lip reading methods are a combination, variation or adaptation of those just described. Whilden and Scally [13] organize their lessons on the articulation movements as conceived by Nitchie—with one "movement" to a lesson—but they are not at all emphasized. Syllable drills are omitted entirely. Section I of each lesson contains (1) a set of sentences based on "movement" words and (2) a story. Section II contains a second set of sentences and either a story or an exercise based on a subject. A chart is used in each lesson as an interest-arousing stimulus, either for the sentence drills or for the exercises. For instance, paper carrots with a "movement" word printed on them could be fed to a pictured rabbit when the child repeated correctly the sentences based on the key words.

The Kinzies [14] combined Nitchie's principles of psychologic theory and Bruhn's organization and classification of sounds in their book for adults. But in their books for children [15] they have made an attempt to prepare material graded to the interests and abilities of children from the first grade to the young adult. The first book is based on informal lessons—the following of commands, simple picture descriptions or stories, guessing games, dramatizations, rhymes and finger plays. The second book is semiformal, the lessons being based on "movements," though these are not stressed. Beside word and sentence drills each lesson consists of a story exercise, rhymes and finger plays. The third book is formally organized and follows the pattern of their book for adults.

Mason [16] developed a series of silent films for self teaching with college students. These were based on a study of the articulatory movements. Though the films were not available outside of her own laboratory they pointed to the possibilities of the utilization of films in teaching speech reading. Morkovin and Moore [17] incorporate in their method some aspect of all of the methods and techniques so far described. Films depicting "life situations" such as a family dinner, a trip to the grocery store, or a birthday party form the basis for the lessons. After a film is viewed once, it is discussed from the standpoint of the situation itself, and of the student's own experiences in relation to similar situations. After further preparation and a second viewing the student is expected to read the conversation of the various characters in the film. Auditory training is an integral part of each lesson. Kinesthetic awareness is developed through exercises in choral speaking. Visual discrimination is accomplished through a study of "movements" found in the vocabulary used in the film.

The teacher will do well to evaluate these various methods of teaching speech reading before she decides on her own methods and techniques. Having done so, she will come to the conclusion, as many of her colleagues before her have, that building a series of lessons on subjects, topics or situations vital and interesting to children is psychologically sound. Learning is expedited when interest is a factor. The unifying effect of a single subject tends to furnish some of the kinds of clues necessary to understanding speech visually. Primary children would enjoy such subjects as "My Dog," "Let's Play House," "Helping Daddy," "Our Trip to the Farm," "Hallowe'en Spooks," "A Doll Party," "The Little Red Wagon," "Cowboy Bill," "Lemonade Stand," "Fire, Fire" and "Out at the Airport," for example. Children in the intermediate grades would like "Black Beauty," "Dude Ranch," "Trip to the Moon," "Let's Play Ball," "Ben Franklin's Key," "Thomas Edison," "Valentine's Day" and "Boys and Girls of Japan" (Holland, Switzerland, and others). High school students are interested in such subjects as "Your Ears and Hearing," "The Good Sport," "Saturday Nite Jamboree," "Football Heroes," "Looking for a Job" and "The President's Trip to ———."

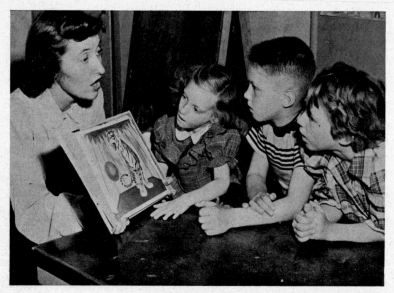

A speech reading lesson developed from a familiar story. Note focus on the therapist's lips.

In each lesson the teacher will try to provide opportunity for the children: (1) To lip read *logically connected* discourse—

well-unified anecdotes, fables or stories—so as to develop synthetic power. (2) To practice lip reading the kind of discourse which is not especially connected—riddles, and sentences related to each other only within the framework of the subject so as to enhance ability to follow a conversation or a class report which might conceivably be disjointed. (3) To become familiar with words that look alike (homophenes) so as to aid in anticipating errors which are legitimate but confusing to the lip reader.

Basing lessons on subjects or topics does not exclude the study of the "movements," but it does eliminate syllable drills. As has been pointed out before, there seems to be no correlation between lip reading of nonsense syllables and general lip reading ability.

The study of the "movements" may be justified and encouraged under certain conditions. A child should be mature enough to have begun reading and to have been introduced to phonics in his regular grade before the study of "movements" is undertaken in speech reading lessons. In fact, hard of hearing children who experience difficulty in learning to read may need a good deal of practice in recognizing the sounds of letters, and blending them into words. This aspect of the lip reading lesson can be nicely correlated with auditory training, and both can be integrated logically with the reading program.

The subject matter of the lesson should not be sacrificed or strained to provide word study or study of a "movement." Word study that grows naturally out of the lesson, or is unobtrusively incorporated into it, can be very effective in helping children understand some of the intricacies of visually perceived language.

The special teacher will go to all of the methods for techniques. She may want to use a movie occasionally as a basis for a lesson. She may use games and devices as suggested by Kinzie and others [18, 19] to increase immediate interest in the drill aspects of the lesson. She may use Nitchie's techniques of rephrasing or developing sentences, and the Jena technique of having the child speak with her for additional clues. She will have informal conversation periods with the children about everyday events or affairs. She will present dramatic readings in which she assumes character parts in order to prepare the children for real dramatizations in which they will participate. There is no limit to the variety of material appropriate for lip reading lessons.

The teacher who prepares her own materials must keep in mind the qualities and characteristics of sentences and stories which make for ease of lip reading. If she is able to construct material that is readily understood by poor lip readers she will have no trouble in varying visibility or structure to make it more difficult for the more adept lip readers. She will then have at her command a useful tool for individualizing instruction within her group. The essential characteristics of sentences and stories are listed and illustrated in tables 2 and 3.

A word should be said about the use of voice in the lip reading lesson. All directions should be given in full voice, and even with amplified voice, so that children are sure to understand what the teacher expects them to do. For a considerable portion of the lesson the teacher may want to use a soft voice which is below the children's threshold for understanding speech auditorily. Sometimes she may want to "turn off her voice" completely. If she has no sound-treated chamber to retreat to, she will have to become versatile in varying the intensity of her voice. She must under no conditions exaggerate her lip movements when she suppresses intensity. The degree of intensity will depend on her aims at a particular moment.

Examples of lip reading-auditory training lessons follow the section on auditory training.

Auditory Training

Hard of hearing children who wear hearing aids for the first time emerge from a relatively quiet world into one of noisy confusion. All around them are sounds which they do not recognize. Often these children express amazement when they first hear water gurgling down a drain, water flushing in the bathroom, the refrigerator's motor humming, and many other household sounds that most people take for granted. The school room

TABLE 2.—*Essential Qualities of Sentences for Speech Reading*

CHARACTERISTICS	EXAMPLES	
	Easier to Read	More Difficult to Read
1. Sentences should be made up largely of visible articulatory movements (see table 1, Chapter 6). The visibility should be distributed evenly throughout the sentence.	The weather has been very pleasant today.	It's a nice day today, isn't it? I like it to be warm but not hot.
2. There should be definite contrast between successive articulatory movements in a sentence.	The barometer has fallen since this afternoon.	It is certain now to turn hot.
3. The more visible the verb, the easier the sentence is to understand.	The clouds drifted slowly across the sky.	The sky cleared in half an hour.
4. Alliteration should be avoided.	The wind blew the man's hat off.	The big storms may spoil our trip.
5. Sentences should be of moderate length. Short ones do not carry enough meaning. Long ones are too difficult to remember.	Five inches of soft white snow fell during the night.	Snow is white. I was surprised when I woke up this morning to see that seven inches of snow had fallen during the night and had drifted across our driveway.
6. Sentences should evoke a definite word picture.	The boys made a snowman out in the back yard.	We have faith in our forecasters.
7. It is easier to lip read a sentence which observes simple order, as subject-verb-object-modifiers, than one which begins with a clause.	I always wear my overshoes when the weather is cold.	If it rains, wear your rubbers.
8. A rhythmic sentence is easier to read than one in which modifiers or parenthetic expressions are interposed between the main parts of the sentence.	I hope that it won't rain tomorrow.	The weather being what it is, I think, after all, that I will take my coat.
9. Verbs in the active voice are easier to understand than those in the passive voice.	The weather will be much warmer tomorrow.	Warmer weather is predicted for tomorrow.

TABLE 3.—*Essential Qualities of Stories for Speech Reading*

| | EXAMPLES | |
CHARACTERISTICS	Easier to Read	More Difficult to Read
1. A story should be logically organized, one sentence leading into the next, the whole being divided into no more than 2 paragraphs and consisting of from 8 to 15 visibly constructed sentences. (Stories for young children should be short but still coherent and have a point.) 2. A story may or may not contain conversation.	*The Barometer Has Fallen* One summer afternoon Jimmy rushed out of the house as fast as he could. He was looking for his father. "Father, father, where are you?" Jimmy called. "I'm in the garage. I'm packing the car so we can go fishing tomorrow," his father shouted. Jimmy ran out to the garage. He was all out of breath and could hardly talk. "What's the matter?" said his father. "Oh, dad, the barometer has fallen." His father was thinking about his fishing trip so he said, "Has it fallen very much?" "Yes," answered Jimmy quickly. "Yes, about 5 feet." "Five feet!" said his father. "I never heard of any barometer's falling 5 feet." "Well, this one has," said Jimmy, "and the mercury is all over the floor."	

3. Biography, history, geography and science make good story material. A single sentence material but poor story material. A single episode or anecdote which has the characteristics noted in 1 and 2 above about a person or event makes a satisfactory story.

4. Inclusion of a great number of proper names makes the discourse more difficult to understand.

5. If a tale or long story is read, it should be phrased in visible language but should not be condensed so as to take the charm out of the original. This type of material lends itself to the seeing-hearing types of presentation, rather than to lip reading alone.

Caught in a Blizzard

Admiral Byrd led several expeditions to the South Pole. His men built their camp on the Great Ice Barrier several miles from the South Pacific Ocean. They unloaded their ships and brought their supplies to camp with dog sleds. Here they built storehouses for their airplanes and for their fuel. They put up tall bamboo flagpoles to mark the trail from ship to camp.

One dark day a dog sled driver started out for camp with a load of gasoline. All of a sudden a blizzard came up when he was 5 miles from camp. Snow began to blow in great clouds and the wind howled fiercely. The dogs became so frightened that they had to be whipped to move on into the storm. The driver could not see the trail or the bamboo poles. His face began to freeze so he put it inside his fur coat for just a minute. In that short time the dogs swerved around out of the wind and off the trail. For a while they were completely lost. The driver forced the dogs back into the wind and at last found a trail pole. From then on, he left nothing to chance. He got off his sled and walked with his dogs safely back to the camp.

Off to the South Pole

Admiral Byrd led several expeditions to the South Pole. He sailed from New York to New Zealand. Then he took his ships to the Great Ice Barrier in the South Pacific Ocean. They arrived in December of 1933. The sun never sets during the month of December at the South Pole. The crew saw many whales in the cold waters along the way. They had their first glimpse of seals and penguins when they reached the Great Ice Barrier.

The long night begins on June 21 and lasts 4 months. The temperature sometimes drops to 83° below zero. Fourteen degrees above zero is the warmest that it gets during the long night. Terrific blizzards rage during these dark months. Admiral Byrd discovered new lands while he was on this expedition. He was the first man to have flown over both the North and South Poles.

is a noisy place, too. Children may be talking, hammering, pounding, scraping chairs, dropping books, sharpening pencils, shuffling feet. The radiator may be banging and hissing, the wind whistling through the trees, the rain beating a tattoo on the window panes and a truck rumbling by, all at the same time. Normally hearing people learn to relegate these sounds to the background, but to hard of hearing children they are the dominant ones when they first put on their aids. How well a child reacts to these distracting, sudden or annoyingly loud sounds, how well he is able to interpret speech in such an environment, how far from the source of speech he can be in a relatively quiet room and still understand what is going on are all matters which have to be studied and evaluated. Since they cannot be deduced from the audiogram, and since the child's response to auditory training is also unpredictable, empiric observation over quite a long period of time may be necessary before an assessment can be made of the child's potentialities for becoming a good listener. A continuing program in auditory training is recommended for poor lip readers, for those who need help in speech and language and for those children who do not easily adjust to hearing aids.

Some children immediately accept a hearing aid enthusiastically and are unhappy if they have to be without it during any of their waking hours. Others are quite reluctant to wear one, and there are some who even refuse to be seen with one. Though they may say that the ear mold hurts, or the cord gets in their way, or that it is too noisy, they may really be ashamed to wear the aid. Forcing children to wear aids against their wills can be very detrimental to a long-range rehabilitation program. In some cases the parents must first be convinced of the value of an aid. Unless they are wholeheartedly cooperative, these reluctant children feel doubly justified in rejecting the aid as an evil instrument. The teacher must acknowledge the children's legitimate discomforts and annoyances, but must also know that familiarity with and use of an aid will eventually eliminate these complaints. She may try to rationalize their fears and dislikes with them, but above all she will have to be ingenious in presenting interesting, meaningful and pleasurable listening experiences, so that these children will really want to hear. They should be introduced to their aids gradually.[20] At first they might wear them only in the auditory training period, and then for a short time in the classroom. They should have the privilege of removing them when they like. Later the time for wearing the aids can be increased until the children wear them continuously.

When a child possesses his own individual aid, both he and his parents should be responsible for its maintenance and care. They should be taught to locate any minor trouble which prevents optimum use of the aid. The preschooler may not be able to insert his own earpiece or regulate the volume control, but he should be able to report when the aid is or is not operating. Even the young child should understand that cords are delicate things and that his aid cannot stand careless or rough treatment.

A child in the primary grades should be able to insert his own earpiece, regulate the volume control, install batteries and report if the aid is not operating properly. Older children should be responsible also for testing and changing their batteries, for inspecting the cords for defects and for cleaning the ear tip. Some older children become very much interested in the structure of a hearing aid and should be given the opportunity to become familiar with its operation, if they so desire.

Auditory training is usually undertaken with children who wear hearing aids, or who are potential users of aids. Children with mild losses, some with marginal losses, and those with normal hearing in most frequencies except the high ones ordinarily do not wear aids. When such children are in the primary grades they too profit from a program of auditory training, even if it is administered without amplified sound. The fact that many books on the teaching of beginning reading emphasize the need of training in auditory perception for all children testifies to its special importance for these children.[21]

If a teacher groups her children for auditory training she will have to individualize instruction within the group, just as she does for lip reading. One child may be able to hear both loud and soft sounds with his hearing aid, and another only the loud ones. One child may be able to discriminate between consonants and vowels, while the next cannot even hear some of the consonants with amplification, much less discriminate between them. The teacher must be cautious lest she get into the habit of accepting the responses of the best hearers as the reaction of the poorest. She must, of course, hold each to his highest potential, but must not discourage a child because he does not succeed as well as another. Using the seeing-hearing approach for the poorer hearers and the auditory alone for the better hearers in exercises requiring fine phonetic discriminations is one way to adjust instruction within the group.

The teacher must have certain equipment at her disposal to carry out an adequate auditory training program. Besides the children's own hearing aids she will need an individual desk type aid for those who do not yet own their own aids, and a group aid for the more severely handicapped, to be used in group instruction. She will want a record player and an abundant supply of recordings of basic rhythms, songs, stories and sound effects.

A few recordings have been specifically designed for purposes of auditory training for primary children.[22-24] Most records, however, have to be selected by the teacher from available commercial lists.[25, 26]

The teacher will find a tape recorder most efficacious in the preparation of materials for her lessons and a stimulating teaching device for use with children who are striving for better speech and listening habits. A knowledge of current children's literature will be most helpful to her, and she will find a picture collection, a collection of noise producing objects, and a mail order catalog invaluable.

In the over-all auditory training program each child is given an opportunity to progress from the easy to the more difficult. In each lesson for primary children, variety may be achieved by including (1) listening to gross sounds, (2) listening to music and song, (3) easy speech discrimination and (4) difficult discrimination if the children have the proper background for it.

Children should, from time to time, be allowed to select what they want to hear, simply because they derive pleasure from it. The program for older children will stress speech discrimination, interpretation and production, but will not entirely neglect listening for pleasure.

A child must first be helped to identify the new sounds he hears through his hearing aid, and then be given practice in recognizing them. There are hundreds of sounds in his environment which he should be encouraged to explore. These sounds are the ones which will serve as the background of his every day living. Their recognition will bring him new but important information about his environment. If he recognizes the ringing of the doorbell as the doorbell at 7:30 in the morning he will be able to react more efficiently than if he thought he heard the alarm clock. These gross sounds are the ones which confuse him when he first puts on his hearing aid. He must learn to sort them out from each other and then he must learn to ignore them when he has to interpret speech in their presence.

Parents can be most helpful in alerting the child to sounds that he would otherwise miss in the home. A child might not hear a parakeet pecking at seeds in his cage, a cat lapping milk, or water dripping from a faucet unless his attention were called to them. Some of the sounds the child should become familiar with in the home are doors banging, telephone and doorbells ringing, dishes being washed and dried, a tea kettle whistling, a pot boiling, meat or eggs frying, corn popping, milk being poured into a glass, noisy chewing, stomping, quiet walking and a clock ticking.

Out of doors a child may miss birds or crickets chirping or wind rustling the leaves in the trees, unless his attention is called to them. He should be encouraged to listen to the sound of raking leaves, shoveling snow, cars passing by, brakes screeching, fire sirens blaring, horns tooting, wind howling and dogs barking.

The teacher and children may explore schoolhouse sounds together. They will hear paper being torn or crushed, typewriters clicking, sewing machines whirring, buzz saws scream-

ing, feet shuffling through the halls and children singing, marching and dancing.

Every time a primary child becomes conscious of a new sound
and reports it to his special teacher he may put a picture of the
sound producing object into his scrapbook. His aim is to get
as many pictures as possible.

Games and devices are used with primary children to provide
fun and motivation for the practice and drill necessary to make
children think more precisely about new sounds they have been
hearing. The teacher may gather 10 to 15 sound-producing objects and place them behind a screen. The poorer hearers may
sit closer to the sound while the better hearers may be stationed
at a greater distance from the source of the sound. The teacher
or a child retires behind the screen. There he piles several
kettles inside each other, pretends to mix a cake with a spoon in
a bowl, drops a cooking pan, pours water from a pitcher to a
glass, operates an egg beater and pretends to dry knives and
forks. Any combination of sounds can be made the basis of such
a lesson. The children are expected to identify and tell about
the sounds as they recognize them. Recordings may be used to
bring sounds to children which are not readily available in the
environment, as animal sounds, farm sounds and city sounds.
Children must at first be aided in identifying the sounds on the
records. Pictures representing the sound source may substitute
for the real objects. Children point to the picture as they hear
the sounds.

Loud and soft sounds should be called to the attention of
little children. Loud stomping can be compared to tip-toeing,
loud clapping with soft clapping, loud music with soft music.
A "hide and seek" game may be played for this aspect of auditory training. While a child steps out of the room, a ball or any
small object is placed in an unusual place but still within sight.
As the child is recalled to the room to find the ball, the teacher
plays loud music or the children clap hands loudly the closer
he gets to the hiding place, and more softly when he veers away
from it in his search. The teacher may play records on which
a train or airplane starts its journey with a loud sound which,

drawing away, grows less and less intense. Children will later have to relate the concept of loudness or softness to their own voices. They may sing or hum quietly at first and then more loudly. Many hard of hearing children do not know how to govern the volume of their voices and must be taught to do so under varying conditions of noise. They must learn to increase the volume in noisy surroundings and decrease it in a quiet environment.

Older children may list the sources and qualities of sounds they hear or have heard. The teacher may get some idea of the kinds of sounds the children are expected to understand, at least at a verbal level, by referring to their readers and to the social science books which they are studying. She must make every effort to give children experiences with the more unfamiliar of these sounds and have the children verbalize about them. They may keep notebooks in which they record the vocabulary related to these sounds as:

The wind sang (howled, whistled) through the trees.
The horse neighed (whinnied, thundered down the road).
The door squeaked (banged, slammed, rattled).

Gross sounds may be variously classified and studied as:

I	II
Sounds at home	Sounds animals make
Sounds on our street	Sounds people make
Sounds at school	Sounds bells make
Sounds at the farm	Sounds machines make
Sounds at the zoo	Sounds water makes
Sounds at the circus	Sounds the wind makes
Sounds in the office	Sounds rain makes

Whatever the organization is, vocabulary building must be an integral part of this aspect of auditory training.

Pitch and rhythm may be brought to the attention of little children through song and bodily activities. Voices of hard of hearing children must be kept flexible and pleasant. They love to sing, as do other children, and need even more practice to keep their voices on pitch than do the normally hearing. Hard of hearing children sometimes find it difficult to understand vocal music because of the variations of the rhythm of speech in the song. Children who can first sing a song will then appreciate listening to it. If recorded songs are used, those with a single voice and single instrument accompaniment are easier to follow than the choral-orchestral type. But before some of these younger children can learn to sing they may have to have specific training in recognizing high and low sounds. The teacher may want to play a low note on the piano, or on a toy xylophone if she has no piano, and let the children indicate "high" by putting their hands above their heads, "low" by stooping to the floor, and middle pitch by placing their arms shoulder high. The teacher may hum a tone and the children may identify it as either low, middle or high. They may be helped by the tactile approach. They may try to match her tone by placing their hands on her face. Even though hard of hearing children do not keep on pitch they should be encouraged to sing. The more they try, the more proficient they will become, especially if they have a little guidance. When the teacher reads a story she may dramatize the characters by speaking in a high voice for a young person or animal and in a low tone for an older person or animal. The children may also use their voices with conscious inflections when they tell stories or imitate animal sounds. Good voice quality and speech patterns will be easier to maintain if children have practice in varying their pitches. Older children like popular jazz songs because of their definite rhythms and their popularity on radio and television. There is no reason why they should not enjoy and appreciate folk songs too, if they are given the opportunities to come to know them.

A rich background of experiences with constant exposure to oral language contributes much to the acquisition of language facility by the hard of hearing child. Skill in auditory discrimination involving speech elements is directly related to the child's knowledge of vocabulary and language. For instance, a young child will not be acquainted with the words *tong* and *thong* or *hone* and *drone* so no purpose is served in asking him to differentiate between them or their component elements. If the teacher thinks that perchance a child is unfamiliar with the word *gown* in the pair of words *gown* and *clown* she might

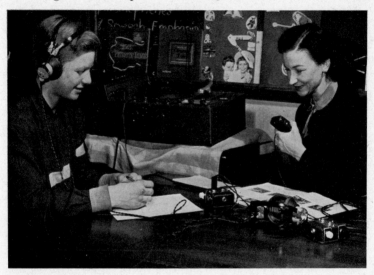

Learning to discriminate among speech sounds is an important part of auditory training.

want to check on the child's experience with wearing a night-gown before she incorporated them into her lessons. No strange word should be used in discrimination exercises, nor should primary children be confronted with isolated sounds in isolated words. They should be presented in context. The special teacher will do well to engage her children in considerable informal conversation so that she may estimate their facility in oral language and speech production in unstructured situations before she plans her program in auditory or speech training.

Discrimination exercises, games or drills involve either recognizing likenesses or differences between words and sounds. The following exercises are suggestive of the types the teacher may use.

Exercises involving vowels: It is relatively easy to identify and recognize vowels.

Differences

(1) Primary children select pictures for the sentences.

> The boy has a *cat*.
> The boy has a *kite*.
> The boy has a *coat*.

> I see a *book*.
> I see a *boat*.
> I see a *bat*.
> I see a *beet*.
> I see a *boot*.
> I see a *bike*.

(2) Older children may identify words containing contrasting vowels by identifying the last word in the sentence.

> How do you *rate*?
> To whom did you *write*?
> Where was the *rat*?
> I know what you *wrote*.

> The farmer has a *goose*.
> The farmer has some *geese*.

Likenesses

Rhyming words, jingles and nursery rhymes bring out the likenesses between vowel elements in words. No attempt is made to point out differences among the consonants in the rhyming words. This is done after the children recognize the likenesses of the vowel sounds.

(1) Primary children complete the rhymes by picking out the correct pictures.

> The little frog
> Sat on a ——.

> This apple you see
> Grew on a ——.

> A great big cat
> Caught a great big ———.
>
> Now let us look
> At this nice story ———.
>
> I saw a mouse
> Run under a ———.

(2) Primary children find pictures which rhyme with a given word.

> *chair* hair pear bear
> *book* (a) cook (fish) hook
> *can* man fan
> *frog* dog log
> *hat* bat rat cat
> *boat* coat goat
> *car* jar star

(3) Older children give all the words that rhyme with a given word.

> *big* pig twig rig wig
> *feather* weather leather heather
> *brother* mother smother
> *walk* talk balk stalk chalk
> *nice* rice slice dice

Exercises involving consonants: It is more difficult to identify, recognize and discriminate between consonants than between vowels.

Differences

(1) Primary children answer simple riddles.

> What sits in a tree, a bird or a worm?
> What do you sit on, a bear or a chair?
> What do you sleep on, a bed or a sled?

(2) Children point to the picture in the pair as the teacher says it.

*sh*oes   *'j*uice

*f*ace   *v*ase

*h*at   *b*at

*m*an   *p*an

Likenesses

(1) Primary children find the pictures for words that begin with a certain sound.

*b*ox   *b*all   *b*ook   *b*eads   *b*uggy

*d*rum   *d*uck   *d*oll   *d*ish

*j*umper   *j*eans   *j*acket

*sh*oes   *sh*irt   *sh*orts

(2) Primary children find pictures of words that end alike: shoe*s*, trouser*s*, stocking*s*, jean*s*; dres*s*, slack*s*, boot*s*, sock*s*, blou*s*e; skir*t*, ha*t*, pocke*t*, shir*t*.

Very good exercises in auditory discrimination for young children are described by Monroe [27] and Ronnei.[28] The former directs her suggestions to the regular classroom teacher, but they can well be used with hard of hearing children who attend regular classes. The latter has specifically designed her manual for hard of hearing children between the ages of 6 to 8 who wear hearing aids. Larsen [29] has prepared sound discrimination lists and recordings for older children in which the consonants are contrasted with one another in paired words. Kelly [30] suggests procedures to be used with high school students and adults.

Two Auditory Training–Speech Reading Lessons

1. For Primary Children

This speech perception lesson is based on a trip to the farm taken by a class of first graders. It can be adapted for a group which has had farm experiences or has seen farm movies. It requires two twenty-minute periods to complete.

Our Visit to the Farm

Materials

(1) Picture of all the farm animals in settings which lend themselves to description, as well as baby animals and their mothers.

(2) Record and Book: *Muffin in the Country,* Young People's Record; *Country Noisy Book,* Margaret Wise Brown (New York, Wm. Scott, Inc.)

(3) Charts (described below, Part II) for review drill for sentences.

Procedure

Part I: Vocabulary

(Teacher uses full voice as do children.)

T.* Let's name all the animals we saw on the farm. (or, Let's name some animals we would see if we went to the farm.)

C. Cows.

C. Horse.

C. Dog, cat, calf, chickens, turkey, rooster, ducks, pigs, bull, etc. *(Teacher places picture of each animal as it is mentioned in a slot chart.)*

(Teacher uses full voice when giving directions.)

T. Now I'll tell you something about them, and you may have the picture if you know which one I'm talking about. Tell me which animal I tell you about.

(Teacher speaks below threshold or at threshold if children do not understand sentences. Children speak words in full voice.)

T. See the brown and white cow.
Where is the horse?
Look at the goose. The goose has a long neck.
The ducks are swimming in the pond.
There are two pigs in the picture.
The cat is black and white.
The lamb is near its mother.
The dog can run fast.
The calf likes to run, too.
The rooster is crowing.

Part II: Phrase and Sentence Drill

(Teacher uses full voice.)

T. Now let's tell where we saw all these animals. (or, I'll tell you where you will have to look to find the animals on my farm.) Tell me what I say.

* *T* stands for *Teacher,* and *C* for *Child.*

(Teacher and children speak below threshold or at threshold. Children may contribute sentences if they like.)

T.   The bull was in the pasture.
      The cows were in the barn.
      The calf was in the barn.
      The dog was in the field.
      The cat was in the barn.
      The ducks were on the pond.

(Teacher now passes out charts and cut-outs to each child. The teacher-made charts, 12" x 18", contain outlines of a barn, barnyard, pond, and pasture. Cut-outs of animals on stiff paper are placed in their proper places on the charts as the teacher reviews sentences in another order.)

Part III: Loud and Soft

(Teacher uses full voice as do children in this exercise in vowel discrimination. The vowels used are o͞o, ah, ow, ee, ŭ, ă, eow. This section emphasizes loud and soft as well as high and low.)

T.   Did you hear the cows moo?
C.   Yes.
C.   No.
T.   Who can moo like a cow?
C.   MOO MOO
T.   How do you think a baby calf would moo?
C.   Moo moo.
T.   Did you hear the dog bark?
C.   Yes.
T.   How does the big dog bark?
C.   BOW WOW
T.   How does the little dog bark?
C.   Bow wow

(Pictures of cow-calf, dog-puppy, cat-kitten, hen-chick, sheep-lamb, etc. are set up in slot chart as children imitate sounds made by all the animals.)

(Children listen with hearing aids turned up to comfortable level.)

T.   Now listen and see if you can tell which animal is talking.
T.   MOO MOO
T.   Baa baa
T.   Peep peep
T.   BOW WOW

(Children point to picture to tell which animal he thinks was talking as teacher goes through entire list.)

Part IV: STORY

(Teacher talks at threshold so that children use hearing and vision to understand story. Teacher pretends to be both Bobby and grandfather by changing position of her head, facing slightly to the right then to the left between each part of the conversation. She does not move her head while speaking.)

T. Now I'm going to tell you a story. This story is about Bobby whose grandfather lives on a farm. His grandfather had a surprise for him. See if you can guess what it is.

SURPRISE FOR BOBBY

T. Bobby went to see his grandfather on the farm. His grandfather said, "I have a surprise for you, Bobby. See if you can guess what it is."
Bobby said, "Is it a new calf?"
"No," said grandfather. "Guess again."
"Is it a new bull?" said Bobby.
"No," said grandfather. "I'll give you one more guess."
"Is it a baby cat?"
"No," said grandfather. "Come to the barn with me and I'll show you."
So Bobby and his grandfather went to the barn. "Look," said grandfather. "Here is your surprise." And what do you think Bobby saw?
(Children may guess at this point.)
Bobby saw five new brown puppies!

(Teacher repeats story or has a child tell story for those who did not understand it the first time. She may ask questions about it instead.)

Part V: LET'S LISTEN

(Teacher uses full voice.)

T. You may look at this book while we listen to this record.

(Teacher plays record, "Muffin in the Country" while children follow in the "Country Noisy Book." Children listen only to identify sounds. After the children are familiar with the record, sections are played in different order. Children identify sounds without looking at the book.)

Part VI: LET'S SING

(Children develop kinesthetic awareness by talking with the teacher.)

T. Now we'll sing a song you all know, "The Farmer in the Dell." I'll
sing it with you.

*(Teacher leads in full voice and children sing with her. Gradually she
reduces her voice and children sing by themselves following her silent
lead.)*

2. For Intermediate Grades

This speech perception lesson was prepared for children in
the fourth grade. "The Farm" is a subject which has been presented at an earlier level more than once. Its familiarity is one
of its virtues. The aim of this lesson is not to teach facts as such,
but to use and review verb vocabulary found in children's
readers, as well as to check on children's ability to recognize and
discriminate between certain phonetic elements, to lip read sentences and connected discourse, and to use the *s* and *z* sounds in
words correctly. It will require 2 thirty-minute periods.

ANIMALS OF THE FARM

Materials

(1) Slot chart for flash cards.

(2) Flash cards containing the names of the following animals which
may be seen on a farm. All the vowel sounds are included in these single
syllable words except *a* and *oi*: goose, bull, goat, dog-frog-hog, sheep-geese-
bees, pigs-chicks, snake, hen, cat-calf-rat-lamb, duck-skunk, bird-squirrel-
worm, cow-mouse-owl, flies, mule-ewe. Flash cards containing the names of
other farm animals as rooster and turkey.

(3) Recording of as many farm animal sounds as possible. Record player.

(4) Rexographed sheet for each child containing words for auditory
training, illustrated in Part III below. Twenty-four cardboard 1″ rectangles
for each child to place over words on sheet.

Procedure

Part I: LISTENING FOR GROSS SOUNDS

*(Teacher uses full voice. Children listen only. Most of them with 40
to 60 db loss will be able to do this satisfactorily.)*

T. I know you have all been to a farm at one time or another but I wonder how many of you have really heard the sounds the animals make.

I have a record here which I am going to play. If you recognize the sound, tell me what it is right away. If you don't know, I'll tell you.

(Record is played twice or as often as necessary to recognize sounds made by lamb, dog, horse, cow, bull, bee, bird, frog, etc.)

Part II: Sentences

A. *Vocabulary for Sentences*

(Teacher uses full voice for giving directions. She calls attention to flash cards in slot chart. Children then read lips and are held to good speech as they repeat words aloud individually.)

T. As you repeat these words after me be sure you use your best *s* and *z* sounds.

T. goose-geese-bees-birds-pigs-dogs-snake-fox-horse-cows-mouse-etc.

T. Now let's see how many different verbs we can use to express the sounds these animals make. Let's begin with the horse.

C. The horse neighs.

C. The horse whinnies.

T. That's correct. We will try to use as many expressive verbs as we can in sentences. I'll give you some sentences. Please repeat each one after me but speak so the others can't hear you. If you don't understand me, please tell me so that I can say the sentence in another way. *(Teacher makes sure that each child can repeat each sentence.)*

B. *Sentences*

(Teacher speaks below threshold. Children may contribute sentences if so motivated. They respond below threshold.)

T. The cow bellowed for her calf.
The dog yipped when the boy stepped on his tail.
The angry bull snorted at the farmer.
The cat purred when I stroked her back.
The mother hen clucked to her baby chicks.
The squirrels chattered to each other in the treetops.
The dog whined because he was lonesome.
The horse whinnied when I gave him some oats.
Did you ever hear a horse neigh?
The lambs were bleating for their mother.
The owl hooted all night long.
The hens cackled when they laid their eggs.

The birds began chirping early in the morning.
The wild goose was honking as it flew over the barn.

C. Sentence Review Drill

(Sentences are read below threshold in another order. If there are several children in the group, the review takes the form of a "spell-down." Children stand in a row. The first child has the first chance. The teacher reads a sentence only once. If the child misses it, he goes to the end of the line, and the next child has the chance to repeat the sentence. If he misses it, he also goes to the end of the line. Each child is responsible for each sentence. The aim is to stay at the head of the line.)

Part III: Vowel and Consonant Discrimination

(Teacher uses full voice.)

T.   In the next part of the lesson we will listen to vowels in words. Turn up your hearing aids so you can hear me comfortably. Here is a paper and 24 markers. When I say a word that contains the key vowel, cover that word. Let's do part "A" now.

A. Vowel Discrimination

(Teacher keeps voice at same intensity as she reads words. Children listen only. Teacher reads down each column.)

A	1	2	3	4	5	6
	aw	ă	-ŭ-	o͞o	ow	ee
	frog	calf	duck	moose	cow	geese
	dog	cow	cluck	goose	mouse	bees
	duck	cat	skunk	horse	house	mouse
	hog	rat	dog	whose	goose	sheep

B		
	1. calf—cat	6. cows—mouse
	2. duck—cluck	7. chicks—pigs
	3. goose—moose	8. bird—chirp
	4. dog—frog	9. skunk—duck
	5. geese—bees	10. hog—dog

B. Consonant Discrimination

(Children who can discriminate consonants listen only. Those who cannot discriminate because of high-frequency deafness may look and listen at first and then try listening only.)

T. Now we will go to part "B." I'll say the two words as they are listed first. Then I'll read them again, but I may reverse the order. Tell me the last word I say.

T. calf-cat
cluck-duck
goose-moose
dog-frog
bees-geese
frog-dog
mouse-cows

Part IV: Connected Discourse

(Teacher uses full voice.)

T. I'm going to tell you a story of some children who were studying about farms. I doubt that any of you fourth graders would give the answer that the last boy did. This story is really a joke. If you don't understand it the first time, I'll tell it a second time.

(Teacher speaks at or below threshold. Poorer lip readers use vision and hearing while good lip readers depend on eyes alone.)

What Is Cowhide For?

T. The boys and girls in Miss Smith's room had visited a farm. They learned that cows were the most valuable of all farm animals. They learned that cows give us milk and cream and meat. They also found out that cows give us hides for our leather shoes and belts.
One day Miss Smith was questioning the boys and girls about the products we get from cows. She said, "Who can tell me what we make from cream?"
One little boy said, "We make butter from cream."
"Fine," said Miss Smith. "What can we make from cow's meat?"
One of the girls raised her hand and said, "We can make sausage out of cow's meat."
"That's right," said Miss Smith. "We can make sausage out of cow's meat. And now, who can tell me what cowhide is for?"
"I know," said another boy. "Cowhide is to keep the cow together."

(Teacher notices reaction to joke to see who understood it. She asks those who know it to retell the story in their own words. Then she re-tells it in her own words, embellishing or revising it to suit the occasion.)

Part V: Word Study—Homophenes

(Teacher and children use full voice. This exercise gives children practice in phonics and sound blending.)

T. You have been listening very well up to now. Let's see how well we can use our eyes for the next part of the lesson. There are several words that look like *duck*. Can anyone think of another word that looks like *duck*?

C. Dug.

T. Correct. Any more? Well, if we can't think of any others let's put our "key" on the board so as to find all the words which look like this one. What sounds like *d*? How do we spell the sounds that look like *ck*?

	—ck	—g	—nk	—ng
t	(1) tuck	(2) tug		
d	(3) duck	(4) dug	(5) dunk	
n				

(Children sound out words and teacher writes them on chalkboard. She does not include any not in the children's vocabulary.)

(Teacher uses full voice.)

T. I'll say some sentences containing these words. Tell me the number of the word which you think I used in the sentence. Say it softly, please.

(Teacher speaks below threshold as do children.)

T. The big ship came into port with the help of a tugboat. (2)
My father shot a mallard duck this fall. (3)
Do you think it is polite to dunk that doughnut in your coffee? (5)
I will have to sew a tuck in my blouse. (1)
We wanted to go fishing so we dug for worms. (4)
You had better duck your head or you will bump it. (3)

T. Now repeat the whole sentence when I give it. *(Teacher repeats sentences in reverse order.)*

Part VI: Let's Sing

*(All sing in full voice. Teacher gradually diminishes hers until chil-
dren follow by watching her lips only.)*

T. How long is it since you've sung "Old MacDonald Had a Farm?" Let's
try it together.

(Teacher may ask a child to lead the song.)

Speech

Speech therapy for hard of hearing children is directed largely
to the correction of articulatory defects and the conservation of
good voice quality. This is not to say that hard of hearing children may not have other speech problems. If a child has a cleft
palate, a serious dental malocclusion, or is cerebral palsied, his
difficulties will be considerably increased. This section will deal
only briefly with the speech problems which result from the
hearing defect itself. There are many excellent texts which describe in detail procedures for diagnosing and treating articulatory and voice problems. In general, the procedures recommended in these texts can be followed with hard of hearing
children with only slight adaptations.[31-35] The teacher will first
have to locate a child's errors before therapy can begin. She
may listen to speech in unstructured situations as suggested
above, make notations of errors and then proceed to a more
formal testing situation in which she uses tests of articulation devised either by others [36] or by herself. The interest of young children can best be sustained by use of a word picture test [37] in
which the sounds appear initially, medially and in the final
position as in *g*irl, wa*g*on, do*g*; *s*oap, era*s*er, bu*s*. The blends
can also be illustrated as in *st*one, *sk*ate, *sp*oon, *sw*im, and in
*dr*ess, *fl*ower, whi*stl*e, bu*ckl*e and but*ton*.

Besides noting the children's articulatory prowess the teacher
must evaluate the quality, pitch and inflection of their voices.
Some older hard of hearing children, especially those with moderately severe losses of long standing, show tendencies to have
monotonous voices with a typical hollow, nonresonant quality.

Some may have too soft voices if they have conductive losses and too loud voices if their losses are of the perceptive variety. Others may exhibit breathy, harsh or excessively nasal qualities which are not necessarily concomitants of the hearing loss. The teacher must determine, or have been aided by medical diagnosis in determining the cause of the voice disorders before she plans the therapy program. The teacher will need, beside the hearing aids and the tape recorder mentioned above, a large mirror when she finds that a child is unable by stimulation through the ear alone to imitate and produce a sound correctly. The vocabulary and language she uses in her lessons should be directly related to children's experiences. Children's progress may be recorded in their notebooks.

Hard of hearing children are generally unaware of their speech disorders, since they speak as they hear. They must be helped to understand and be convinced of the desirability of correct and clear articulation and good voice quality. Everything else being equal, a child who is internally motivated to strive for better speech will make gains far beyond those of a child who is indifferent about his speech. Primary children respond to the immediate, and will usually work diligently and happily for a small reward whether it be social approval of the teacher or a star on a piece of paper. The immediate reward is not enough for the older children. They need to know what their long range goals are, but they should not feel overwhelmed by too complicated a plan. When one goal has been reached, new ones may be set up. In this way the children have a feeling of accomplishment but are still challenged and stimulated to move forward to new conquests. For the correction of an articulatory defect, the teacher may follow the general procedure suggested below.

(1) Present many times—not just once—clear auditory-visual-tactile impressions of the sound through the hearing aid, and in the context of the word. The child should be able to identify and recognize the correct production of the sound by hearing alone, if possible, by vision alone, and by the seeing-hearing method.

(2) Present only one new sound at a time. Teach this sound in isolation:

(a) By direct auditory-visual-tactile stimulation. The child imitates the teacher after being given an adequate pattern.

(b) If this fails, by contrasting the child's incorrect production with the teacher's correct production. The teacher imitates the child in order to contrast incorrect placement of articulators with the correct one.

(c) If this fails, by working from analogy of a sound whose position is similar, as from *sh* to *s* for a tip-up *s* or from *ee* to *z* for a tip-down position.

(d) If this fails, through tongue exercises which tend to strengthen control of the tongue position sought.

(e) If this fails, by manipulating the speech organs.

(3) Incorporate the sound in simple well known words which contain no other difficult sounds, as *r*ow, *r*un, *r*ide; *s*ave, *s*even, *s*uit; wal*k*, boo*k*, bi*k*e.

If the child is unable to produce such combinations readily, because he falls back into old incorrect habits automatically, the sound may be placed first in nonsense syllables, each of which becomes the basis for a word.

(4) Teach the blends containing the sound both initially and finally as *cl*own, *cr*ayon, *qu*een, *cl*ean; bu*ckle*, chi*cken*, wal*ked*, six.

(5) Use the words in children's original sentences and in conversation, making the child responsible for the detection of his own speech errors. If at this stage the child makes errors in agreement of tense, as "Daddy walk to work," be sure that the child understands the reason for adding the *s* or *ed* to this form of the verb.

(6) Encourage the child to strive for correct and automatic use of the sound in all his speech.

Exercises for helping hard of hearing children with their voice problems have been suggested in the preceding section on auditory training. Some children will show spontaneous improvement in the quality of their voices when they begin to wear hearing aids. Others will improve after receiving auditory training and a few will need added help of tactile-kinesthetic training.

Some suggestions for developing control of voice through the tactile-kinesthetic approach follow.

(1) Teacher hums on a basic pitch: middle C, B or B-flat below middle C. Child feels muscle sensations as teacher produces soft resonant hum. Child imitates this basic pitch.

(2) Child imitates teacher's basic pitch using syllables m——a, m——a, ma; m——aw, m—aw, maw; m——oe, m——oe, moe. The same pitch is always used.

(3) Child imitates teacher's hum one octave higher, and proceeds to produce syllables (as in 2 above) on this pitch. Child imitates teacher's hum one-half octave higher and proceeds to produce syllables on this pitch.

(4) Child then begins on lower pitch and glides to higher pitch and vice versa, imitating teacher.

(5) Child learns to imitate any intermediate pitches presented by teacher through use of the tactile-kinesthetic clues.

(6) Child speaks a simple sentence on basic monotonous pitch.

(7) Child varies pitch pattern using normal variations of pitch. Changing emphasis of words in a sentence is a good cue for varying pitch and volume.

RECAPITULATION

Hard of hearing children are so much like their hearing brothers and sisters in the development of their ability to communicate orally that they should receive their education in the regular elementary school. In face-to-face conversation with one other person most of these children will experience little inconvenience in communication, but in group discussions and conversation and in situations where the source of sound is beyond their hearing range they will experience considerable difficulty unless they have developed skill in interpreting speech from combined visual auditory stimuli. Early detection of the loss, and early use of amplified sound are important in alleviating their communication problems, and in forestalling poor speech habits. Parents play an especially vital role in the educative process. What they think about the child's loss will greatly influence the child for good or for evil.

In the regular classroom, seating arrangements for these children should be flexible. The teacher and their classmates will speak clearly but without exaggeration, because they know that sight as well as hearing are important to understanding what they say.

The special teacher will guide these children in the development of skill in lip reading and auditory discrimination according to their capacities, and she will guide them toward better speech. She will have gathered pertinent information about them and will plan their special program according to their needs. If she teaches several children with different needs in one group, she will individualize instruction within the group. She will always try to guide parents to greater understanding of the children's problems, and she will try to guide the children to a better understanding of themselves.

REFERENCES

1. JOHNSON, WENDELL, DARLEY, F. L. AND SPRIESTERBACH, D. C.: Diagnostic Manual in Speech Correction. New York, Harper & Bros., 1952.
2. VAN RIPER, CHARLES: A Case Book in Speech Therapy. New York, Prentice Hall, 1953.
3. BACKUS, OLLIE: The use of group structure in speech therapy. J. Speech & Hearing Disorders 17: 118–122, June 1952.
4. UTLEY, JEAN: How well can you read lips? 1946.
5. ——: A test of lipreading ability. J. Speech & Hearing Disorders 11: 109–116, 1944.
6. DiCARLO, LOUIS AND KATAJA, RAY: Analysis of the Utley lipreading test. J. Speech & Hearing Disorders 16: 226–240, September 1951.
7. BRUHN, MARTHA: The Mueller-Walle Method of Lipreading for the Deaf. Lynn, Massachusetts, Thomas P. Nichols & Son, 1924.
8. ——: The Mueller-Walle Method of Lip Reading for the Hard of Hearing. Boston, M. H. Leavis, 1947.
9. ——: Elementary Lessons in Lipreading. Lynn, Massachusetts, Nichols Press, 1927.

10. BUNGER, ANNA: Speech Reading—Jena Method. Danville, Illinois, The Interstate, 1932, 1952.

11. NITCHIE, EDWARD: Lipreading Principles and Practice. New York, Frederick A. Stokes, 1912.

12. STOWELL, AGNES, SAMUELSON, ESTELLE AND LEHMAN, ANN: Lipreading for the Deafened Child. New York, Macmillan, 1928.

13. WHILDEN, OLIVE AND SCALLY, AGATHA: Newer Method in Speech Reading for the Hard of Hearing Child. Westminster, Maryland, John William Eckenrode, 1939.

14. KINZIE, CORA AND KINZIE, ROSE: Lipreading for Deafened Adults. Seattle, Washington, Cora, Elsie Kinzie, 712 Securities Building.

15. —— AND ——: Lipreading for Children (Books I, II, III). Seattle, Washington, P. O. Box 2044, 1936.

16. MASON, MARIE: Teaching and testing lipreading by the cinematographic method. Volta Review 44: 703, December 1942.

17. MORKOVIN, BORIS AND MOORE, LUCELIA: Life Situation Speech Reading through Cooperation of the Senses. Los Angeles, University of Southern California, 1949.

18. FABREGAS, MINNIE AND SAMUELSON, ESTELLE: A Treasure Chest of Lipreading Games. Washington, D. C., Volta Bureau, 1939.

19. MACNUTT, ENA: Hearing with Our Eyes. Washington, D. C., Volta Bureau, 1953.

20. RONNEI, ELEANOR AND PORTER, JOAN: Tim and His Hearing Aid. New York, Dodd, Mead, 1951.

21. McKEE, PAUL: The Teaching of Reading. New York, Houghton-Mifflin, 1948, pp. 151–154.

22. Sounds Around Us. Scott, Foresman & Co., 433 E. Erie St., Chicago 11, Illinois.

23. UTLEY, JEAN: What's Its Name (workbook and two recordings). Urbana, Illinois, University of Illinois Press, 1951.

24. WHITEHURST, MARY: Two Records and Manual for Auditory Training. New York, Hearing Rehabilitation, 330 E. 63rd St., New York 2, New York.

25. EISENBERG, PHILIP AND KRASNO, HECKY: A Guide to Children's Records. New York, Crown Publishers, 1948.

26. TAUSSIG, ELEANOR AND STONER, MARGUERITE: Phonograph records for the young child. Volta Review 51: 355, August 1950.

27. MONROE, MARIAN: Growing into Reading. Chicago, Scott, Foresman, 1951, pp. 110–139.

28. RONNEI, ELEANOR: Learning to Look and Listen. New York, Bureau of Publications, Teachers College, Columbia University, 1951.

29. LARSEN, LAILA: Sound Discrimination Lists. IN Hearing and Deafness, a Guide for Laymen (Davis, ed.). New York, Rinehart Books, 1947.

30. Kelly, James: Clinicians Handbook for Auditory Training. Dubuque, Iowa, W. C. Broun, 1953.

31. Backus, Ollie: Speech in Education. New York, Longmans Green, 1943.

32. Irwin, Ruth B.: Speech and Hearing Therapy. New York, Prentice Hall, 1953.

33. Johnson, Wendell et al.: Speech Handicapped School Children. New York, Harper & Bros., 1948.

34. Van Riper, Charles: Speech Correction Principles and Methods. New York, Prentice Hall, 1947.

35. West, Robert, Kennedy, Lou and Carr, Anna: Rehabilitation of Speech. New York, Harper & Bros., 1947.

36. Templin, Mildred: A study of sound discrimination ability of elementary school pupils. J. Speech Disorders 8: 132, 1943.

37. Bryngelson, Bryng and Glaspie, E.: Speech Improvement Cards. Chicago, Scott, Foresman, 1941.

Bibliography

General

Backus, Ollie: Speech in Education. New York, Longmans, Green, 1943.
——: The use of group structure in speech therapy. J. Speech & Hearing Disorders 17: 118–122, June 1952.

DiCarlo, Louis and Kataja, Ray: Analysis of the Utley lipreading test. J. Speech & Hearing Disorders 16: 226–240, September 1951.

Ewing, Irene: Lipreading and Hearing Aids. Manchester, England, Manchester University Press, 1946.

Eisenberg, Philip and Krasno, Hecky: A Guide to Children's Records. New York, Crown Publishers, 1948.

Irwin, Ruth B.: Speech and Hearing Therapy. New York, Prentice Hall, 1953.

Johnson, Wendell, Darley, F. L. and Spriestersbach, D. C.: Diagnostic Manual in Speech Correction. New York, Harper & Bros., 1952.

—— et al.: Speech Handicapped School Children. New York, Harper & Bros., 1948.

Mason, Marie: Teaching and testing lipreading by the cinematographic method. Volta Review 44: 703, December 1942.

McKee, Paul: The Teaching of Reading. New York, Houghton-Mifflin, 1948.

Templin, Mildred: A study of sound discrimination ability of elementary school pupils. J. Speech Disorders 8: 132, 1943.

Utley, Jean: Factors involved in teaching and testing lipreading ability through the use of motion pictures. Volta Review 53: 657–659, 1946.

Van Riper, Charles: A Case Book in Speech Therapy. New York, Prentice Hall, 1953.

——: Speech Correction Principles and Methods. New York, Prentice Hall, 1947.

West, Robert, Kennedy, Lou and Carr, Anna: Rehabilitation of Speech. New York, Harper & Bros., 1947.

Auditory Training Materials

Brown, Margaret W.: Muffin in the Country (YPR), Country Noisy Book. Boston, New York, Wm. R. Scott.

Kelly, James: Clinicians Handbook for Auditory Training. Dubuque, Iowa, W. C. Broun, 1953.

Larsen, Laila: Sound Discrimination Lists. In Hearing and Deafness, a Guide for Laymen (Davis, ed.). New York, Rinehart Books, 1947.

Monroe, Marian: Growing into Reading. Chicago, Scott, Foresman, 1951, 110–139.

Ronnei, Eleanor: Learning to Look and Listen. New York, Bureau of Publications, Teachers College, Columbia University, 1951.

—— and Porter, Joan: Tim and His Hearing Aid. New York, Dodd, Mead, 1951.

Taussig, Eleanor and Stoner, Marguerite: Phonograph records for the young child. Volta Review 51: 355, August 1950.

Utley, Jean: What's Its Name. Urbana, Illinois, University of Illinois Press, 1950.

Whitehurst, Mary: Manual for Auditory Training (with two recordings). Hearing Rehabilitation, 330 E. 63rd St., New York 2, New York.

Lip Reading Materials for Children

American Hearing Society: New Aids and Materials for Teaching Lip-Reading. Washington, D. C., American Hearing Society, 1943.

Bruhn, Martha: Elementary Lessons in Lipreading. Lynn, Massachusetts. Nichols Press, 1927.

Fabregas, Minnie and Samuelson, Estelle: A Treasure Chest of Lipreading Games. Washington, D. C., Volta Bureau, 1939.

Kinzie, Cora: Lipreading for Children (Books I, II, III). Seattle, Washington, P. O. Box 2044, 1936.

MacNutt, Ena: Hearing with Our Eyes. Washington, D. C., Volta Bureau, 1953.

Stowell, Agnes, Samuelson, E. and Lehman, Ann: Lipreading for the Deafened Child. New York, Macmillan, 1928.

Whilden, Olive and Scally, Agatha: The Newer Method in Speech Reading for the Hard of Hearing. Aberdeen, Maryland, Hartford Printing Co., 1929.

Lip Reading Materials for Adults

BRUHN, MARTHA: The Mueller-Walle Method of Lipreading for the Hard of Hearing. Boston, M. H. Leavis, 1947.

BUNGER, ANNA: Speech Reading—Jena Method. Danville, Illinois, The Interstate, 1952.

KINZIE, CORA AND KINZIE, ROSE: Lipreading for the Deafened Adult. Seattle, Washington, P. O. Box 2044.

MONTAGUE, HARRIET: Lipreading Lessons for Adult Beginners. Washington, D. C., Volta Bureau, 1945.

MORKOVIN, BORIS AND MOORE, LUCELIA: Life Situation Speech Reading through Cooperation of the Senses. Los Angeles, University of Southern California, 1949.

NITCHIE, EDWARD: Lipreading Principles and Practice. New York, Frederick A. Stokes, 1912.

NITCHIE, ELIZABETH: Advanced Lessons in Lipreading. New York, Frederick A. Stokes, 1923.

——: New Lessons in Lipreading. Philadelphia, Lippincott, 1950.

ORDMAN, KATHRYN AND RALLI, MARY: What People Say. New York, The Nitchie School of Lipreading, 1949.

Speech Material for Children

BRYNGELSON, BRYNG AND GLASPEY, E.: Speech Improvement Cards. Chicago, Scott, Foresman, 1941.

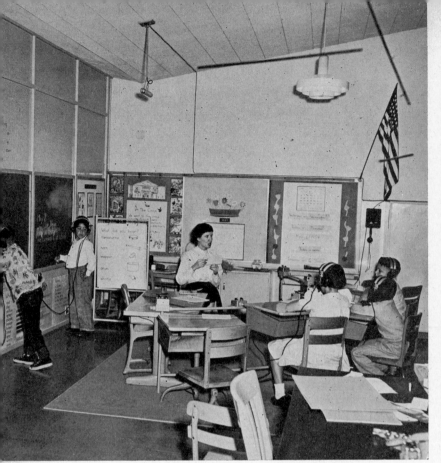

hoto courtesy A. M. Brooks Co., Los Angeles

8

Education of Children with Severe and Profound Hearing Losses

INTRODUCTION

THE children whose education will be discussed in this chapter are those whose language and speech fail to develop spontaneously because of severe hearing impairments which have existed from birth, from early infancy or from before the time when language emerges. It is not unusual for alert parents to suspect deafness in such children when they are only babies, for they conspicuously do not respond to the louder sounds about them, nor do they learn to respond to their names at an age when normally hearing children do.

Though the emotional impact of the discovery of deafness may be temporarily devastating to parents, the early discovery itself should be regarded as a blessing in disguise, for then and there the education of the child and parents can begin. To be effective, this education must be a continuing process for the parents as well as for the child. As the child grows and develops, as his needs change, so must the parents' understandings and appreciations be increased. The deaf child will need all the help that his teachers and both parents can give him along the difficult educational road he will travel.

Except in situations where familial deafness exists, relatively few people have contact with children who have been deaf since birth, since the incidence of such deafness is not very great. For every 1000 children in regular elementary and high schools [1] there are only seven children in schools for the deaf.[2]

Thus, it is possible that many people may go through life without actually meeting a deaf person face to face. The consequence of this lack of contact results in widespread ignorance about the problems of the deaf. A not unusual reaction of a seemingly intelligent stranger upon striking up a casual conversation with a teacher of deaf children is one of confusion, as witness the following episode:

Stranger: And what do you do?

Teacher: I teach deaf children.

Stranger: I suppose you can read Braille, too.

Teacher: No, I teach deaf children, not blind children. The deaf can see, but they can't hear.

Stranger (after an embarrassed pause): Of course, I should have known better. The deaf and dumb talk with their hands, don't they?

Similar situations occur time and time again. And since parents are people, they cannot be expected to know instinc-

tively or learn overnight the complications and frustrations, or
the joys and satisfactions that go with being parents of a deaf
child. They will need time to absorb information and grow
wise with their children. All the suggestions made in the previous chapter on the role of parents also apply to the parents
of the deaf child. But these parents will need supplementary
information to help them understand the special problems
which very limited hearing imposes.

Establishing and Maintaining Communication

A deaf baby reacts to his early environment much as does a
baby who hears. He cries when he is hungry or uncomfortable,
and he smiles when he is pleased. The deaf baby learns to
interpret his mother's moods as she takes care of him, but he
does this mainly through visual and kinesthetic senses. He can
tell by her actions whether she is in a hurry or upset, and he can
also sense when all is well. He feels it in his muscles and he
may see it in her face. Since he hears no language, his mother
will have to communicate with him largely through her facial
expressions at first. Of course she will talk to him continually
as she does to any other child. Catching the child's glance frequently and speaking with her eyes as well as with her lips will
encourage the child to watch her face and to respond to her
pleasure and joy in him. What better time has she to do this
than when she is looking down at him in his crib, when she is
strolling him in his buggy, when she is feeding him or bathing
him. Later, when the need for a "no" arises, the child will learn
to interpret this expression along with others of surprise and
disapproval.

There will be a great temptation, especially as the child grows
older and more mobile, to gesture to him; for instance, to direct
him to drink his milk with a drinking motion, or to come with
a beck of the finger. Wise parents will avoid even natural gestures, for if a child gets into the habit of watching the hands
for information, he will cease to watch the face. This means that

retraining of both parents and child will have to take place later. It is always more difficult to try to break down unfavorable habits than to avoid forming them in the first place. As a substitute for the natural but somewhat formalized gestures just mentioned, the mother will have to demonstrate frequently what she means. If she wants the child to remove his shoes at bedtime, she may take off one of them for him. Then holding the shoe in her hand near her mouth she can say, "Now you take off a shoe," with an encouraging glance at the one shoe on the child's foot. Or if she wants the child to come to sit down for dinner she may go to him with a glass of milk and say, "Come now, we're going to eat. Sit at your table." Later, lip movements alone begin to take on meaning because they have been associated countless numbers of times with objects or activities, and the child learns to watch face and lips. It is reported that a child as young as one year of age has actually learned to read lips.[3] Every time a deaf child's attention is directed to a person's face, that person should be ready to say something to the child, if only: "You're mother's big boy," or "Are you having a fine time with your blocks?" If a deaf child is to learn to speak he must see speech continually. An oral atmosphere is indispensable to learning to speak.

The child's gestures, however, should not be repressed, for he has no other means of expressing himself in the beginning. Later, his fumbling attempts at speech may be substituted for his gestures, and then his best speech efforts must be encouraged. This means that parents must ever be aware of his capabilities and speech accomplishments. At first the parents may have to be clever guessers of what the child wishes to communicate, if he is not to be utterly frustrated. If a child tries to express a seemingly important thought, need or desire which is not immediately understood, it is a good idea to lead him from room to room or from object to object in search of the thing he has in mind. If he just wishes to communicate some friendly but unimportant piece of information and he is not really understood, the listener should at least look interested and make some kind of verbal response however innocuous it be. Every effort should be made to understand and respond to the child's attempt at communication, for if he knows he has an attentive audience he will feel free to communicate. If he doesn't, he may soon learn to withdraw, or if he is an aggressive child, to throw a tantrum out of sheer frustration at not being understood.

The tactile sense of the deaf child will be an important one for him in learning speech. The mother can help the deaf baby become aware of sound through vibration by talking to him when she is holding him in her arms. He will feel the vibrations in her chest and head as she talks or sings to him, especially if she directs his attention to them by placing his hand on her cheek or chest. She can do this as she cuddles him before she puts him to bed or when she feeds him after his bath. She can encourage him to use his own voice if she hears him babble. The baby's hand may even be placed on his own cheek to let him "hear" himself.

Parents of deaf babies can begin early to watch for signs of hearing in their children. Though it is possible to test the hearing of infants by means of the psychogalvanic skin response test, many parents will not have access to this test. One hearing test is not sufficient to diagnose or evaluate the hearing of young children. Little children who seem quite deaf as infants may be found later to have trainable residual hearing. Therefore it is very important that parents explore their children's hearing informally.[4]

Though young deaf children may respond reflexively to loud sounds close to their ears by blinking their eyes or even turning their heads, they soon lose interest and pay no attention to meaningless sounds. The mother may, however, from time to time, test the baby's startle-responses to sound by calling to him when he is not looking, or she may shake his rattle close to his ear. She may notice his response or lack of response to these and various other loud sounds around him. She may also sing or talk close to his ear while he has his hand on her face, though she should exercise caution lest her breath tickle the child and annoy him. She should not cease to subject him to sound even though she is doubtful that he hears anything at all. Since deaf children are more apt to hear low frequency sounds it might be well for the father to talk and sing to the baby too. For the two or three year old who is sitting on the mother's or father's lap as they are looking at picture books together, the parent may say the words into the child's ear, if he does not already wear a hearing aid, as he points to the pictures. The child should be encouraged to vocalize in response to these auditory impressions as well as to tactile impressions. Whenever a child consciously or unconsciously makes use of his voice, parents should show satisfaction and pleasure. If the child does not become aware that he has a voice he will become a silent child.

Hearing Aids for Deaf Children

After parents have explored the hearing of their children at close range, they may wish to introduce sound through use of a hearing aid, under the guidance of a trained worker. The age at which this is done depends somewhat upon the responsiveness of the child to amplified sound and upon his maturity. Some seemingly quite deaf children respond to hearing aids successfully at the age of two or three. The more profound the loss, the more difficult it is to make the children aware of sound and to make sound meaningful. Unless sound can have significance, children will not enjoy having a hearing aid clamped on their ears. The first introduction to the aid must be pleasurable and not forced. Often a child as young as two becomes interested in watching television, whether for good or for bad. An earphone connected to the set can be provided for him. Parents may wear dummy headsets, or bona fide ones if they wish, over a period of several weeks while they listen to television. Without any urging the child will soon consider it routine procedure to wear a headset himself. After he has become accustomed to such listening, a small desk type amplifier may be used during the evening story hour and at mealtime after the child is old enough to join the family at the table. It is entirely possible that after such procedure has established the child's willingness and even eagerness to hear, he may have his own individual aid. This means that parents will have to adjust the aid and supervise its upkeep until he can do so himself. He may never be able to interpret language and speech with his aid alone, but he may hear such sounds as bells, vacuum cleaners, shouts and car horns. This amount of sound is considered sufficiently important to warrant wearing a hearing aid by many older deaf children for interpretation of the environment.

Unfortunately it is necessary to teach little children the limits of the noise which they can make. They may love to pound on their mother's kettles with a spoon while wearing their hearing aids, but the neighbors upstairs won't appreciate the din. In one breath the child is told to, "Hear! hear!, Listen! listen!" and in the next to "Stop! stop! stop making that awful noise!" Such training will have to be tempered with judgment.

Many little children discover their voices only when they begin to wear a hearing aid. Increase of babbling is frequently a concomitant of wearing an individual aid. It is agreed by most people who work with little deaf children that early awareness of sound enhances and reinforces the child's later appreciation of it, and that any hearing that a child has should be utilized at as early a date as possible.

Discipline

Parents tend to guide their children in the light of their own personalities, adjustments and customs. They impose certain inhibitions on their children and define for them what they may and may not do, what they must do and what they must not do. This they usually do through liberal use of verbal controls followed by rewards and praise, or isolation and punishment. When parents use a great many negative commands, their children tend to be highstrung and nervous; when they use restricting commands, children tend to become inhibited; when parents issue conflicting commands, constructive behavior diminishes. Oversolicitousness on the part of the mother prevents development of self-reliance and fosters immature behavior which may manifest itself in submissiveness or aggressiveness, depending on individual reactions. Parents' conscious or unconscious rejection of the child seriously disturbs the child's sense of security. On the other hand, children who feel secure in their parents' love for them, who live in a democratic and permissive atmosphere and who are given responsibilities within their capabilities are more likely to be cooperative, self-reliant and, later, popular in school.

Since one cannot talk to, or reason with, a deaf child, parents have to try to show by example the kind of behavior expected of him. In families where there is a good deal of good natured rough-housing, pushing and slapping, the deaf child will sometimes carry over this type of behavior to his playmates, who in turn will resent it. How can a deaf child know that such activity is to be frowned upon? He cannot be punished for what is accepted at home, but he will soon be isolated by other children if the pushing and hitting is not stopped outside as well as in the home. Likewise, in families in which physical punishment is the mode of control, the child will learn that hitting is an acceptable form of behavior. Parents may have to re-evaluate their actions and controls if they do not want their children to emulate their bad habits.

Some parents, in order to placate a deaf child who is fussing at home or in public, indulge him to keep him quiet, instead of trying to get at the root of his behavior. Some anticipate every whim and desire in order not to come to grips with a possibly rebellious child. These families will soon be tyrannized by their children. There is just as much necessity for guiding the deaf child into acceptable standards of behavior as any other child.

Understanding parents realize that a deaf child passes through the same stages of physical development as other children. He likes to tear paper, scatter contents of waste baskets, climb and run. He also goes through stages of stubbornness, negativeness and mischievousness just because he is a child. His parents are careful not to confuse typical childhood behavior with behavior that results from limited hearing. If a mother decides that she does not want the contents of all her dresser drawers emptied onto the bedroom floor, it is not enough for her to say "no, no" to the child. She may show the child and also say, "You mustn't do this, but you may empty this drawer. *This* is yours." Or, shaking her head say, "You mustn't tear up the telephone book, but you may tear this. *This* is yours." Unless a deaf child is shown what he can do, he won't know what is expected of him. It is not enough to say "no." A constructive statement must always be added. This really gives the child a sense of security even if it thwarts his pleasure of the moment, for he knows the limits within which he can function.

A sense of security is also fostered by a consistency in the requests directed to the child from day to day by the various members of the family. If the child is allowed to scribble on the walls on Monday and Tuesday but not on Wednesday because his mother's patience suddenly wore thin on Wednesday, the child will have no notion of why he is being disciplined. Likewise, if the mother tells the child that it is time to go to bed and the father says he can stay up for another half hour, the child will be confused about the conflict between the parents, and in turn will manifest a definite sense of insecurity if such type of behavior is often repeated by the parents.

Parents who are well adjusted to each other, and who accept the deaf child at face value with love, will be able to surmount the communication difficulties they encounter in trying to help their children to normal standards of behavior. It is important that deaf children assume increasing responsibility for self-discipline as they grow up. They cannot afford to be different from other children if they are to be accepted in a group of their peers.

Parents as Teachers

Parents who avail themselves of the opportunity to learn about deafness and its effects on the development of their children are usually whipped into a frenzy of training and teaching activities. They learn that the early years are important, and therefore feel that they must not waste a single minute of the child's time. Many a conscientious parent sadly discovers that efforts to teach his child end in failure. What is first an eagerness on the part of parents may turn into tension when the child does not respond according to the rules set up by the experts. The transfer of tension to the child will inhibit his learning. Thus, a vicious circle of thwarting and frustration is set up. If this occurs, parents must seek further guidance before attempting to help the child.

Parents and teachers alike sometimes fail to take into account the importance of maturity in the learning process. When a child's muscular development and coordination reaches a stage where he is able to walk, he walks with a little practice. When a child is able to use his smaller muscles, to string beads for instance, he will be able to string beads. Forcing a child to walk or string beads before he has sufficient muscular maturity to perform such tasks is but a waste of effort on the trainer's part. Few parents would seek to urge a child to learn to walk prematurely. Forcing a child to put puzzles together, to match certain geometric shapes or to solve an arithmetic problem before he had developed sufficiently intellectually would be just as unrealistic as expecting him to learn to walk before he was ready. Therefore parents must become astute in arranging learning situations within the child's capacities. With greater experience and added maturity a child may learn a certain task, like putting on his shoes or putting puzzles together, with less formal practice than if he had been drilled and drilled in the task before he was ready to do it. Success is important in keeping a child's interest. If he fails continually, his zest for learning is killed. By the same token a task which is too easy dampens a child's enthusiasm for learning. Perhaps it should be reiterated at this point that parents will achieve greater success in training if they guide and teach as a matter of course in the total contacts with the child rather than by the clock.[5]

Little children do not react favorably to formal teaching, and if parents decide to act like teachers for 15 to 30 minutes during the day, the parent-child relationship can easily be destroyed. Parents will, from time to time, have periods of depression about the slowness, the seeming hopelessness of what they are trying to do. They must take heart, and realize that a minor miracle will eventually be performed—teaching a deaf child to talk. By not expecting too much of their children too soon, by not forcing learning, but by relaxing and by demonstrating what is desired and desirable, parents can guide their children to become increasingly self-reliant and to develop good habits of communication. Parents will, of course, have to plan on going to school with their children, since there is much for all to learn until the time when the children themselves have finished their formal education and are self-sustaining adults.

Where Deaf Children May Go to School

The education of deaf children in the United States has been traditionally institutional in nature. From 1817 to 1869 when the first day school was established in Boston, all deaf children attended residential schools.[2] At first the growth of day schools was rather slow. In 1945, 70 per cent of deaf children still received their education in public residential schools, but by 1955 about 60 per cent did. The trend to send children to day schools is likely to continue. One of the recommendations in the Platform of the Mid-Century White House Conference [6] urges, in regard to furthering healthy personality development through the schools, that local boards of education accept full responsibility for planning and providing adequate educational programs and services including special services to meet the needs of children with physical and mental handicaps, and that the state departments of education assume responsibility for leadership in realizing such an objective. Emphasis on the early diagnosis and education of deaf children has also contributed to the growth of day schools. Many parents hesitate to send three-year-olds away from home to school, though a few residential schools admit children at that age.

Deaf children who attend public residential schools live in dormitories or cottages under the supervision of matrons or house parents during the school year, and return to their homes during vacation periods. Tuition, room and board are free in state public residential schools for residents of the state. Children share work and play experiences, and build strong school spirit loyalties and friendships during the years they spend together.

Residential schools provide for organized religious education and vocational training. The methods of instruction vary with the schools. Twelve of the 75 schools in the United States use only the oral method of instruction, but most maintain some manual classes for the children who do not seem to be successful in learning speech.[2] Except in the oral schools, out-of-class communication is usually carried on by means of signs or finger spelling. The greatest number of these schools admit children at the age of six. Fourteen schools offer complete secondary programs while 12 offer training through the Junior High School level.

It is difficult to make generalizations about the residential schools, for some are small (5 children) and some are large (490 children); some are ancient and some are modern; some are very traditional in their approach to education and some are cognizant of modern trends.

Parochial schools and classes are maintained by the Roman Catholic Church and by the Lutheran Church. Private schools and day classes together with the denominational schools serve about 9 per cent of the children in schools for the deaf. The children are taught by the oral method in these schools. Private schools maintain small classes which allow for a good deal of individual instruction. They admit children at a very early age, some at 16 or 18 months. Tuition costs in these schools vary considerably.

Public day classes are generally housed in a regular school where the deaf children may or may not have daily contacts with hearing children. This depends upon the philosophy of the school system, and the cooperative spirit among the entire school's staff. The children in many of these classes have opportunities to associate with the hearing children in sports, playground activities, Girl and Boy Scouts, all-school projects and in art and gym classes. A few may take all or just part of their academic work with hearing children. Some of the larger day schools are housed in their own buildings, and during the school day the deaf children are as completely segregated from children who hear as those in residential schools. The younger children are generally transported free to and from school daily, while the older children use public transportation as soon as they are able to do so. The children who attend these schools are taught by the oral method almost exclusively. Some day schools admit children as young as 2 and 2½ and most admit them between the ages of 3 and 3½. Only a few require the child to have reached the age of 5 or 6 for admission. Close ties are maintained with parents in many of these schools through parent-teacher organizations. Parents are kept abreast of the progress of their children and are encouraged to help children at home to use the language they learn in school. Most of these schools offer training through the eighth grade. Generally, children who attend high school are expected to go to the regular high school, but in some cities special classes are maintained for deaf children at the high school level.

As with the residential schools, it is difficult to generalize about day schools. The smallest center gives service to 3 children, the largest to 540. They vary in physical plant, in philosophy and in the quality of instruction, just as the residential schools do. If a parent is considering moving to a community with a school for deaf children, so that the child may live at home and enjoy the security of parental care and affection, it would be wise to visit several schools before making a final decision as to where to locate.

Gallaudet College in Washington, D. C., is the only college for the deaf in the world. It has a preparatory course for students who are not fully qualified for the college course, as well as a college course. Classroom instruction is given by means of combined use of signs, manual alphabet and speech. Many deaf persons have also attended and have been graduated from regular colleges throughout the United States.

The Teacher of the Deaf

Her Competencies and Qualities

The deaf child's teacher must be a very versatile person. The nature of her job requires that she have a ready knowledge and considerable skill in many areas before she can efficiently teach children with very limited hearing.

1. She should have a good understanding of the principles of child development, so that she, like parents, can arrange learning situations within the child's levels of maturity.

2. She should be well informed about modern educational procedures and curricula in the regular elementary schools. She will have to be expert in adapting them to the appropriate conceptual and verbal levels of deaf children of all ages, since educational retardation is almost inevitable with these children.

3. She must, of course, be thoroughly grounded in the details of the communicative process as discussed in the previous two chapters. This requires, as a prerequisite for teaching speech, a well trained ear, an ability to analyze errors instantly and correct faulty production. She must be familiar with the various methods of language teaching that have been devised for instructing deaf children.

4. She must be cognizant of the various speech perception techniques referred to above. She must be able to adapt these techniques to the varying needs of each deaf child. Most important, she must appreciate the interrelationships between lip reading, auditory training, teaching of speech and language and the subject matter fields. She must be able to correlate and integrate them all in her teaching. The degree to which she accomplishes this will determine her skill as a teacher.

5. As a background she will have to know about the ear: its structure, function and abnormalities, so that she can deal intelligently with otologic reports.

6. She must be able to test hearing with the audiometer and interpret responses to the more complex clinical speech-hearing tests.

7. She should be familiar with the structure and operation of hearing aids, so as to be able to do elementary trouble shooting in case of a breakdown of her equipment.

8. She should be conversant with the latest developments for displaying speech visually, as typified by the Sonograph which is an adaptation of the first instruments used to record "visible speech" electronically.[7]

9. She should have an appreciation of the use and interpretation of psychologic tests for deaf children, so that she may understand their intellectual capacities and emotional and social adjustment problems.

10. She should have a background in the history of American education of the deaf, so that she may gain insight into, and be better able to evaluate present-day problems.

11. She should know a good deal about the adult deaf in our society so that she can guide her children intelligently into good personal and vocational adjustments.

12. A knowledge of human behavior and adjustment will help her deal more competently with the children she teaches. She will want to know specifically about each child in her class in regard to his behavior at home, his reactions to parents and siblings, and to his neighborhood.

13. She will have to be a guide for parents in their spiritual struggles against disappointment and uncertainty throughout the years. She will also want to help them to encourage their children to achieve to their highest capacities.

14. She will have to be a first-rate public relations agent, for she must lead the children's classmates, teachers in the regular school, administrators, guidance workers and employers to a better understanding of deaf children.

15. The teacher of the deaf will have to be a stable and well-adjusted person with a high tolerance for frustration. She should be dedicated and willing to work for more than money. Her job is a difficult but rewarding one.

The Children She Teaches

Though this teacher may possibly be expected to teach the hard of hearing, the children most frequently found in her classes will have either severe or profound losses.

Ray and Larry are two children who may be considered representative, though not necessarily typical, of these latter two groups. They both entered a small public day school at the same time when they were four years old. Neither had any speech or oral language when he began going to school. Each was an only child with better than average intelligence as measured by the Ontario School Ability Test.[8] The great difference between them lay in the amount of hearing each possessed, and inevitably in their personalities.

Both of Ray's parents were profoundly deaf. They had been educated in residential schools, one in a private, and one in a state school. They communicated by signs with Ray, with friends and with relatives. Ray's mother read lips very well and spoke quite intelligibly, but his father was reluctant to talk at all. He held a good job as a skilled worker in a local manufacturing plant. The parents realized early that Ray had a hearing loss but assumed that he was deaf. His aunt who lived in the neighborhood suspected that he had some hearing and urged his mother to take him to a clinic for an evaluation of his hearing when he was three and a half. Here Ray responded to loud gross sounds but not to language. It was recommended that he enter a special class for children with limited hearing. His audiogram at five and a half is shown in figure 1.

Ray himself was a nicely adjusted child. He learned language rapidly after he entered school, though special techniques were used to teach it to him until he went to high school. His voice had natural inflections and his speech was intelligible, but he had some difficulty in incorporating the sibilants into his speech. A group hearing aid was used for all of his instruction. Ray never resorted to signs at school, though he used them at home.

Ray's parents were not interested in buying him an individual aid. Presumably, because they were deaf, they underestimated the value he would derive from one. They always had excuses for not buying one. Their house needed painting one summer; the next year they had to have a new car; and the next they had to take a trip to a National Park to use the car! Finally, when Ray was twelve, he got his own hearing aid, but he still wears it reluctantly.

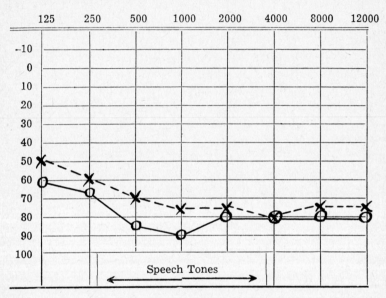

FIG. 1.—Ray's audiogram—considered reliable at age five and one-half. In this and the succeeding audiogram, O = right ear, X = left ear.

Ray's pleasant personality made him popular among his classmates. By the time he was in the second grade he went to art and arithmetic classes in the regular grades. In the fourth grade he also participated in the sports class and spelling class. He eventually joined the Scouts and participated in all their activities. By the time he was in the sixth grade he went to regular classes for all his work except language arts and social studies. He still required a good deal of help in vocabulary and in developing reading skills and comprehension, but he made steady and excellent progress so that he could enter into the complete regular academic high school program. He returned to the special class teacher for only two periods a week for tutoring in English and for lip reading and auditory training during this time.

He is now 18 years old, in his junior year in high school and receiving grades a little better than average. These he honestly earns. He belongs to the biology club and is active in sports. He wants to go to college and will undoubtedly be able to do so successfully because of his fine adjustment and strong drive to succeed. Nobody who meets Ray for the first time thinks of him as being deaf, for he speaks well and uses fluent language. As a result of a properly tailored program he has the characteristics of a hard of hearing person rather than those of the profoundly deaf child his parents thought him to be.

If Ray had attended a large, rather than a small elementary school for the deaf, he would undoubtedly have been placed in a special class within the school. These classes, variously designated as "acoustic classes" or "auditory training classes," emphasize the training of residual hearing. The children who, like Ray, attend them make relatively fast progress in learning language and speech.

If children like Ray are not sent to special classes or schools their stories may not have so happy a theme as his. Many such children have been discovered sitting in classes in the regular schools. They are regarded as stupid because their speech and language are fragmentarily or only partially developed. They become retarded and neglected children.

Larry lived with his mother and father, a successful businessman, in an upper middle-class neighborhood where there were no other little children. The parents discovered his hearing loss when he was about two, and asked for help from the local teacher of the deaf. They were only half-hearted in receiving guidance and soon ceased to come for conferences. His mother also failed to complete a correspondence course for parents of deaf children.

Larry pretty much had his own way at home. If his fancy was taken by a red wagon with silver wheels, he got it. He was a resolute little fellow by the time he entered school. He de-

manded a good deal of attention from children and teacher by
pushing, poking and acting the clown. He was quite at ease with
adults and enjoyed being with them more than he did with his
classmates.

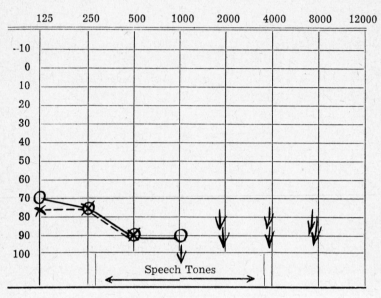

FIG. 2.—Larry's audiogram at age six.

Larry was profoundly deaf (see figure 2). When he was six,
his parents bought him the most expensive hearing aid they
could get. While it remained a novelty he wore it faithfully,
though he was never aware of the loud squeals which emanated
from it when his earpiece got too close to the microphone.
Sometimes he was oblivious of the fact that it wasn't even
turned on. He refused to wear the stronger group aid in class
work because he insisted he could hear better with his own.
Persuasion finally induced him to try the group aid but he never
learned to identify more than gross sounds and two vowels
over it. His voice was well placed and his speech was quite
intelligible despite his profound loss.

He learned language and speech only because he had a skilled teacher who was more resolute than he. Larry liked the easy things in life, and learning language was not one of them. Fortunately, he was very fond of nature and the out-of-doors. At his family summer home he learned to swim, to run a motor boat and to sail. He collected rocks and insects. When these interests were challenged he worked like a beaver, so he did manage to learn some speech and language. Through his skill in sports he eventually achieved status with the other boys in the school, and they were glad when he was one of the team. He learned gradually how to become popular without being a pest.

Larry never went out to regular academic classes in the elementary school though he did attend art and sports classes. He read lips readily when he knew what the conversation was about and if it was conducted on his level of language understanding, but he did not understand language well enough to be placed satisfactorily in a regular class with his own age group. Larry is now of high school age and though he attends classes in physical education, manual arts and art for half a day in the regular high school, he still receives instruction in language from the special class teacher. He wishes now that he could go to college, but his level of achievement will not permit this. His early background of poor work habits, combined with his profound deafness, mitigated against his achieving academic success commensurate with his intelligence. Larry has shown aptitude in art and is skilled in the use of his hands. Undoubtedly he will be able to find a job as a skilled workman. His training now is being directed toward vocational interests and in helping him to form better work habits.

A child who has as profound a hearing loss as Larry generally learns speech and language slowly and laboriously. Factors which contribute to a deaf child's educational success are: (1) his intelligence, (2) his personal and social adjustment, (3) the age at which his education begins, (4) the help he receives around the clock, other than from his teachers and, perhaps as important as any other, (5) the skill with which he is taught.

THE SCHOOL PROGRAM

The Early Years: The Organization of the Classes

There is no general concensus among educators of the deaf as to the best type of organized educational program for young children with severe hearing impairments, though there is wide agreement that early education is desirable, if not imperative in order to forestall extreme educational retardation and to make use of the crucial years between two and six for learning language. As a consequence, age for admission to nine of the 75 public residential schools, seventy-six of the 163 day schools and classes, and forty-one of the 53 private schools was 3 years or less in 1954.[2]

One need only peruse the literature of former years to be convinced that this development is rather recent. It is true that an interest was aroused in nursery schools and kindergartens for deaf children by the turn of the 20th century, but this interest waxed and waned throughout the first three decades and only since the 1940's has it seemed to be an abiding one.

The pioneer ventures in educating young deaf children were not publicly supported. They were beacons, however, which shed their lights afar and have left their marks on our schools of today. The first oral preschool for deaf children justifies its fame. It was organized in 1883 in Chicago by Miss Mary Mc-Cowan.

Children as young as three were soon admitted to the Voice and Hearing School for the Deaf. Miss McCowan felt that the deaf child should be encouraged to investigate everything in his environment, and through use of the "natural method" should secure a knowledge of language which would enable him to proceed through the curriculum of the regular school with a distinct advantage.[9]

Alexander Graham Bell, also in 1883, established a private school in Washington, D. C., to which both hearing and deaf children were admitted at the age of four and a half. They played together, but the deaf were instructed separately. Socialization and contacts with the normally hearing were stressed here. After Bell was no longer able to devote his attention to this school, it was carried on using Bell's methods of teaching speech for several more years by Miss Anna Schmitt, a kindergarten teacher whom Bell had employed in his school.[9]

In 1888 the Sarah Fuller Home for Little Children Who Cannot Hear was opened near Boston, Massachusetts. It accepted children of ages from three to six. The school was disbanded during World War I and reinstituted as a home teaching service in 1927. Itinerant teachers now go from home to home instructing parents and children alike. The guidance of families is stressed in this service.[9]

After World War I several chapters of the American Hearing Society, led by the New York League for the Hard of Hearing, began experimental programs for young children on a clinical part time or full time basis. Since World War II other service organizations, as the Junior League and the National Society for Crippled Children and Adults, have been instrumental in starting preschool classes, some of which later became publicly supported. The growth of programs in universities and hospitals as adjuncts to clinical services has been quite spectacular in recent years. Here young children are tested, parents are guided, and children are taught on clinical bases. A few clinics also maintain regular classes for deaf children. These programs are usually held in conjunction with training teachers, otologists, psychologists and social workers.

In large residential and day schools where the annual enrollment of three-year-olds reaches 10 to 12 children, nursery classes for deaf children are the usual rule. Children with severe and profound losses attend school for the entire day—or part of the day—eating, napping, playing and learning informally under the direction of trained nursery school teachers and teachers of the deaf. In many of these classes the nursery teacher is in charge of the social group, while the teacher of the deaf is responsible for helping those children who are mature enough to receive specialized training in speech.

Many variations of this sort of program may be observed

throughout the United States. In some schools, parents or volunteer workers take the place of the trained nursery school teacher when funds are not available for the hiring of two teachers for a small group. In other schools, only traditionally trained teachers of the deaf are employed for nursery school classes. Here each teacher is entirely responsible for all aspects of the program for her own group of six or seven children. Unless the staffs involved are well versed in nursery school procedures, these programs are not likely to be as effective as they could be.

In public day schools where it is not possible to control enrollment by selection of pupils and where the number of three-year-olds admitted annually varies from one to three or four children—too few to establish a class—other means must be devised to meet the needs of the children and still carry out the objectives of preschool education, of which socialization is a most important aspect. In order to provide such opportunity for three-year-olds, parents are encouraged to enroll children in established nursery schools for hearing children. Some of these schools have been reluctant to accept deaf children for fear their programs would be disrupted by the presence of a child who was different. Such a situation demands the full cooperation of the teacher of the deaf and of the parents with the nursery school teacher. As soon as she learns how to communicate with the child, her fears are usually allayed. She will find that the deaf child can adjust to routine, and will fit nicely into her group.

If there is no nursery school in the community, the parents may try to make provisions for contacts with other little children in the neighborhood. This may mean that several children, hearing and deaf, will play together in an oral atmosphere under parental guidance.

The lone three-year-old deaf child may spend several half-hour periods during the week with the special teacher, getting acquainted with her and the other children in her room. At the age of four the child usually becomes eligible for enrollment in a kindergarten, if the school system maintains kindergartens.

He attends school for only half a day, as do other four-year-olds. The child remains in the kindergarten for the activity and play periods and goes to the special class teacher during the singing and story hour periods.

If possible, it is desirable to send only one little deaf child to any one kindergarten. This arrangement does not place a burden on the regular teacher, and it also gives the child every opportunity to become acquainted with the other children in the class. If two or more deaf children are enrolled in a regular kindergarten they tend to gravitate toward each other, thereby retarding the socialization-integration process.

Another adaptation of procedure in the day school program is one in which the teacher of the deaf takes her class of six or seven five-year-olds to the regular kindergarten for an hour or so a day, where she is able to guide and direct not only her pupils but the other members of the group into better social relationships. She also uses the time for informal teaching of language based on the children's activities in the kindergarten.

Still another adaptation possible in a day school program is one in which the five-year-old deaf child who has attended a nursery school for deaf children for several years, and who has ability to read lips, comes to the school for the deaf for part of the morning for special instruction. He goes home early for lunch and rest, and then to the kindergarten in his own school district for the afternoon program. This enables him not only to become acquainted with deaf children, but to make friends with children of his neighborhood.

Each program of each school and each community tries to meet the needs of the children it serves. Consequently there can be no unanimity of program, though the aims and objectives of all should have a common ground. A good nursery program for deaf children provides for: (1) socialization of the child, (2) informal learning through direct experiences in an enriched physical and social environment, (3) establishment, informally, of communication through the eye by means of lip reading, and through the ear by means of amplified sound and (4) guidance of parents.

Today, parent education is an integral part of most nursery school programs whether they be publicly or privately supported. In some schools, two-way vision screens or mirrors are provided so that parents and other observers will not distract the child or cause unusual abberations in their behavior. In other situations parents are encouraged to participate in the play program, and even teach some of the children, though not their own. Regular evening meetings which both parents attend are often part of the program. Some nursery schools will not accept children unless the parents agree to enroll in the course set up for them.

The Program for Children From Three to Six

The nursery school as it is known today is truly an educational institution. While it is not to be considered simply as a

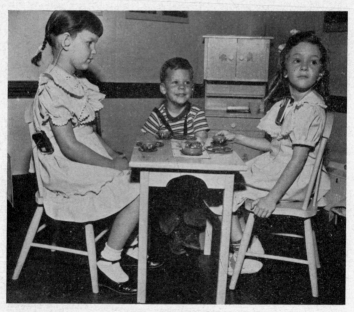

Play activities may be used as purposeful learning experiences.

place where children go for custodial care, neither is it expected to replace the home. It supplements the home by furnishing a rich environment favorable to learning. Play is a highly effective method of early education, so practice in the nursery school is keyed to children's preoccupation with play. The kindergarten program is an extension of the nursery school. It is organized to fit the life needs of children as they grow and mature.[10]

In modern schools for the deaf the program for children with very limited hearing follows the philosophy of the regular nursery school. Unfortunately, in the past some teachers of deaf children have neglected to take into consideration the characteristics of little children and have subjected three-year-olds to methods of teaching designed for six- and seven-year-olds. The tendency to teach toward the handicap rather than to teach the child has caused the focus to be placed incorrectly on formalized instructional procedures. As teachers gain a little understanding of child growth and development many of these poor practices have been, or are steadily being eliminated. Each child must be taught first as a child and then as one with a hearing loss. The teacher must be aware of the individual differences among her group. One child may be physically and mentally mature, but socially inept; another may be mentally a bit slow and physically uncoordinated; another may have a visual handicap besides his hearing loss; another may be well developed physically, mentally and socially.

It is not possible to state specifically what any particular child will accomplish during his first year in school, or in any year thereafter. The levels of accomplishment designated in the following discussion are only indicative of what a child might achieve under favorable circumstances. One child may require two years to complete what another does in half a year. The steps he follows will be those outlined in table 1, but the rate at which he proceeds will be his own.

Every phase of the nursery program presents excellent opportunities for situational lip reading. During the out-of-door play period a teacher may be helping a three-year-old up the ladder to the top of the slide. She takes his hand, and catching his glance as he waits his turn to go up she says, "Up, up, up you go!" and as he is poised at the top for the downward slide, she

TABLE 1.—*Outline of Language and Speech for Children 3, 4 and 5 Years of Age*

Level	Characteristics	Language: Receptive	Language: Expressive	Instruction In Speech and Language
3 year old	Can play cooperatively. Enjoys outdoor play. Likes doll and block play.	1. Child learns to appreciate social meaning of oral communication. 2. Language concepts are built around everyday nursery school experiences. 3. Children learn that things have names.	May depend on gesture to communicate ideas. Vocalizes in free play periods with expression of emotions. May imitate a few words if he has residual hearing.	Teacher talks in sentences. She accepts any attempts at communication. There is no formal instruction in speech or language. Teacher explores child's hearing ability.
4 year old	Can play in group. Enjoys active outdoor play. Likes easel painting and coloring. Enjoys puzzles, looking at books. Enjoys rhythmic activities.	1. Receptive stage predominates through speech reading. 2. Language concepts are built about activities: running, games; holidays: Christmas, Halloween, Thanksgiving, Easter; dramatic play, story telling, excursions. 3. Child recognizes names of pets, toys, foods, furniture, dishes, clothes, parts of body, everyday means of transportation. 4. Child begins to appreciate meaning of pronoun "I."	Child begins to name objects by attempting speech of simple words. Partial speech is used more than complete speech. Single words are used to express complete thoughts or ask questions. Some simple sentences attempted as: I ran. I fell. I laughed.	Teacher talks in sentences. Readiness for articulation is explored: Blowing games Rhythmic games Finger plays Good voice is encouraged and emphasized. Child may learn to recognize printed symbols in sentences. Imitation is encouraged. Child is not held for exact speech.

TABLE 1.—*Outline of Language and Speech for Children 3, 4 and 5 Years of Age (Continued)*

Level	Characteristics	Language: Receptive	Language: Expressive	Instruction In Speech and Language
4 year old		5. Readiness for reading is established through: (1) story telling, (2) language of everyday affairs.		
		6. Concepts of passage of time—today, yesterday, and tomorrow are developing.		
		7. Colors are recognized on lips.		
5 year old	Enjoys group activities. Likes learning. Likes to make things and experiment with materials. Enjoys stories and dramatization.	Receptive stage continues. Language experiences are based on: 1. Excursions into neighborhood. 2. Playing house. 3. Celebrating holidays. 4. Storytelling. 5. Planned activities relating to homes and school experiences. Vocabulary includes all categories on 4-year level plus tools and growing things.	Sentence sense established this year, though partial sentences still predominate. Uses pronouns I, you, we: (a) with past tense: (1) of *intransitive verbs:* ——ran, ——fell, coughed, ——went ——. (2) *transitive verbs:* saw ——, ——made ——, ——found——. (b) with present tense: ——have——, am——, ——is ——, like——.	*Speech* Individual instruction is begun in speech. Child can imitate all speech sounds in syllables except more difficult combinations. Child can produce blends: bl (blue) kt (walked); tt (went to). Child differentiates between p, b, m; t, d, n; k, g, ng, as initial or final sound in words.

263

TABLE 1.—*Outline of Language and Speech for Children 3, 4 and 5 Years of Age (Continued)*

Level	Characteristics	Language: Receptive	Language: Expressive	Instruction In Speech and Language
5 year old		Concepts of time are related to everyday experiences.	Uses expressions: I thought. I forgot. I love you. May I have some water? Come.	Sentence length breath is developed. Rhythm is expected in sentence production. *Language*
		Concepts of number 1–4 or 5 are established.	Uses some adjectives and adverbs as: new, big, small, up-down.	Rules are not presented formally.
		Adjectives describing common characteristics are beginning to be understood.		Child may be helped to classify some words under captions: WHO and WHAT.
		Concepts of place are established through understanding of prepositions in, on, under, etc.		Child is encouraged to include verb in sentences.
		Reading is established through: 1. use of charts based on group experiences, 2. individual experiences, 3. dramatization of stories, 4. following printed commands.		Child should begin to recognize printed symbols if he does not already do so.
		Understands questions. Did you——? Have you——? Who——?		

264

says, "Down, down, down you go!" Every time she encounters a child's glance she says something apropos of the situation. It might be "Let's fill the pail with sand," or "Please give me the shovel." Or, as she is helping children learn to share toys, she may say, "John has the wagon now. You may have the wagon after a while." Again, to another child, "Here is the rabbit. The rabbit is in his house. You may give the carrot to the rabbit." The teacher always speaks in simple, clear and correct sentences.

When a little group goes for a short walk in the neighborhood and gathers mementoes of the trip—dandelions in the spring or leaves in the fall—the teacher names the namable objects the children have collected. Children also begin to learn elementary safety rules on these trips. The teacher says, "Wait for me. Take my hand when we cross the street."

Indoors, during the lunch period, children are helped not only to accept new and different foods which they may have refused at home, and to eat quietly, but they also see the names of the foods, dishes and utensils on the teacher's lips as she eats with them during the lunch period: "Do you want more milk, Sue?" "The potatoes are good," "Shall I help you with your meat, Don?" "You may have more carrots, Beth," "This is your napkin, John."

During the rhythm period, children gain better coordination and an extensive verb vocabulary. Many little deaf children must be taught not to shuffle when they walk. Activities like marching call their attention to the need for picking up their feet. They run, tiptoe, walk like elephants, hop like rabbits and beat drums. All these activities are verbalized by the teacher during each rhythm period. At this time the children also become conscious of vibrations of piano, tomtom or drum. The teacher plays or beats out marching, running or walking rhythms. The children terminate their marching, running or walking activities as the music or drumbeat stops. When a teacher notices that a child responds quickly to piano vibrations at a distance, she may suspect that he has some hearing. This child should undoubtedly be wearing a hearing aid if he does not already do so. The other children follow the lead of this child until they also can recognize independently the presence or cessation of vibrations. Later, when children are learning speech, their knowledge of vibration or lack of it will stand them in good stead.

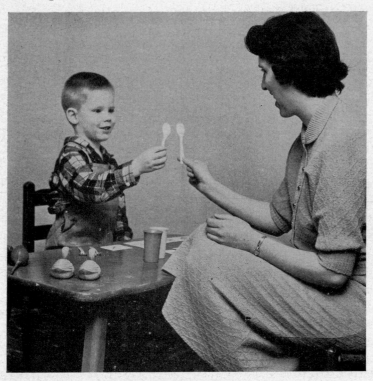

Learning to match objects, colors, textures and pictures helps the young deaf child focus his attention, refine visual perception and build associations.

Three-year-olds enjoy jumping, running, clay modeling, doll play and block building. All these activities are rife with language possibilities. Through use of art materials and dramatic play with dolls and blocks, children's imaginations can be developed. The teacher can also draw inferences about the child's personality and social relationships by observing him at play.[5]

Birthdays and holidays at first have little meaning for deaf children. If there is a celebration of each child's birthday at the time it occurs, the significance will eventually become established. Time is still an unknown dimension to little children, and especially to those who cannot hear. No effort is made at this level to teach passage of time with the calendar.

Even though there is no formal instruction, constant daily repetitions in the same situations, using the same language again and again, cannot fail to impress on the children the significance of the spoken word. The children may soon learn to respond to oral directions because they anticipate them in specific routine situations maintained in the daily program. They also learn to respond to their names. Many three-year-olds learn to recognize in lip reading the names of several of their favorite toys, and the names of some of the other children in the class. This is the beginning of language understanding. Children must have much exposure to simple clearly spoken language before they can be expected to respond in speech. If they do attempt to imitate, and many do, their fumbling efforts should be eagerly accepted, and the children should be made aware of the teacher's pleasure in their attempts. The teacher may want, however, to explore the children's readiness for speech by first having them imitate her large bodily movements in a follow-the-leader game, then finer movements through the use of finger plays,[11] and finally the movement of the lips and of some visible tongue movements. All of this is accomplished in game activities of short duration. If she finds a child who is especially adept at speech imitation she may encourage him to articulate an attempted word such as *ball,* or *doll,* or *bike.* The teacher encourages speech but does not teach it formally at this age level.

The lives of four-year-old children are still largely oriented to active vigorous play. They play more planfully than three-year-olds and with considerable imagination. They now enjoy being members of groups. They are intent on exploring the world about them. They like books, painting, coloring and putting puzzles together.

It is very important that there be an abundance of planned activities and experiences for the deaf children at this age. Though some four-year-olds are capable of considerable concentration, most have not developed the ability to attend to any task or game or experience for a very long time. The experiences therefore should be of short duration and related to the children's immediate interests. Planned experiences are used for language development and are so arranged as to accord opportunities for repetition of vocabulary as well as for development of new vocabulary and language understandings. For instance, children might make simple paper hats for a birthday party, or Indian bonnets for a war dance. At another time they might make cocoa for a party. They could make baskets and fill them with grass in anticipation of the Easter rabbit's arrival.

Short excursions into the neighborhood to see a neighbor's new puppy, to the park in winter to slide down a hill, in summer to sail boats, or the corner store to get carrots for the rabbit may become very profitable language experiences. Parents should be encouraged to take their children to the zoo, the community playground, the airport and to a farm. The children should not be denied an enrichment of experience through extended trips, but the immediate environment should be the basis for the child's directed language experiences in school. Until the vocabulary and language connected with the immediate is well established and stabilized through varied repetition, the remoter aspects of the community may be deferred as school experiences.

Four-year-olds who have been in school for a year quickly add many new words to their lip reading vocabularies. They learn to recognize the names of the more visible objects about them.

Toys: car, blocks, train, truck, doll, drum, airplane, ball

Animals and pets: dog, cat, bird, rabbit, chicks, ducks

Dishes: cup, fork, spoon, plate, glass, sauce dish

Clothing: coat, cap, shoes, dress, blouse, shirt, sweater, tie, socks, pants

Food: milk, ice cream, cookies, potatoes, meat, bread, carrots, cocoa, soup, sauerkraut

Schoolroom equipment: book, easel, piano, paints, light, colors, scissors, paper, hearing aid, table, chair, shelf, desk

These words are important only as they relate to the child's ability to understand them in the context of a sentence. Too many teachers and parents speak to deaf children in single words. This gives the child an erroneous impression of the use

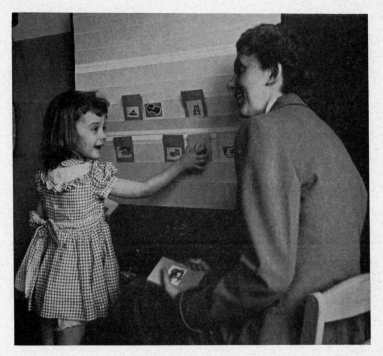

Speech reading of nouns. Note child's focus of attention on the teacher's lips.

of words. Words are used to express ideas. Ideas are best expressed by the use of sentences. If children have had the opportunity to see words used in sentences, they will begin to respond to specific commands not directly connected with a situation. For instance, a child may come in from out-of-doors and drop his coat on the floor in his hurry to get to his favorite truck before some one else does. The teacher approaches him and says, "Your coat is on the floor. Hang up your coat, please." If by chance he does not understand, she may take him to where the coat is and then repeat her directions. She should continually ask some child to fetch an object for her. "Please get the ball for me," "I want the drum and the drum sticks. Who will get them for me?" "Where is the big doll? Bring the doll to me." Four-year-olds do not enjoy sitting down at a table for a stilted formal drill in which the teacher speaks and the child points as in "Show me a drum," "Show me a top," "Show me a ball," but he does enjoy using his ability to read lips in a meaningful situation calling for activity.

Stories can fire the imagination of little deaf children as well as children who hear. New language concepts can be introduced and developed through dramatization. Stories at this level must be simple and graphically illustrated.[12] The teacher will have to adjust her story telling techniques considerably, for she cannot talk and show pictures at the same time. Children should first have an opportunity to see each picture on a page before the teacher begins to talk. The teacher may use various conditioning devices with her group so that they look at her face when she speaks. She may use a short cardboard pointer no more than six inches in length which she may shift from the picture to her mouth as she begins to talk. Closing the book momentarily or covering the page with a piece of cardboard may also signal the fact that the children are to look at the teacher's mouth. When a certain mode of telling stories has been established, children can derive tremendous benefit and pleasure from the story hour. An interest in books is fostered through the telling of stories.

Time is beginning to have a bit more meaning for children of four. They should begin to develop a concept of *yesterday, today* and *tomorrow,* tentative though it may be. A picture record of daily activities drawn by the teacher may be kept on a large 40″ x 40″ calendar which contains no numerals. The drawings may frequently be referred to as "Yesterday we went to the park," "John is sick today," "We will not come to school tomorrow." As each day passes it is crossed off the calendar.

Through painting and coloring activities the children learn to identify and recognize the names of colors through lip reading. In these activities deaf children should be given full freedom to express themselves and to experiment with materials. Adult standards must not be imposed upon them. If the children are asked only to copy pictures or color outlined forms such as balls, birds or cars, their sense of free expression will be deadened. Deaf children have so little means of expressing themselves that they should be encouraged to use drawing and painting as a means of conveying thoughts to others. Through their original drawings the teachers may gain insight into their personalities, their intellectual capabilities and into how they perceive the world.[13]

At this stage children can begin to appreciate the meaning of the pronoun "I." They are still largely egocentric, as are four-year-olds who hear. They like to show off their own possessions, their drawings and other accomplishments. They point to themselves continually when referring to "I," "mine" or "me." During the daily conversation period or the show-and-tell period, children may be expected to use the language they have been gradually absorbing. They may use only single words to express whole sentences. The child may say "fe" when he means "I fell." The teacher may help him to say "I fell." With enough repetitions of this kind the child will begin to use the pronoun "I" in simple sentences.

After a visit to the park the children may want to report, "We saw some ducks" though they may only say "du du du," indicating numbers of ducks. They may draw pictures of the ducks as their contribution to the experience, and the teacher may supply both the oral statement, "We saw some ducks," and the printed form if the children are ready for the latter.

Only after children have a firmly established, rather extensive vocabulary in lip reading (50 to 100 nouns understood and used in conjunction with 10 to 15 verbs) should they be introduced to the printed symbol. They should be able to identify and recognize a circle, a square and a triangle, and to recognize differences and likenesses in such readiness exercises as described in publisher's materials and in Lassman's and Monroe's books.[14, 15]

A few of the more mature children will be able to engage in

this sort of activity at the end of their fourth year, but many will not be able to do so until they are five and perhaps six. The children who are ready to respond to the printed symbol will profit from having the furniture and other objects in the classroom labeled, though no effort is made to have the children match or identify these symbols independently.

Four-year-olds with trainable residual hearing may become rather adept at imitating speech. They may spontaneously try to repeat what the teacher is saying to them. Use of their muscles seems to reinforce their memories of the visual form of the word, and it should be encouraged. As soon as any child gives evidence that he wants, and tries, to talk he may be helped to produce a word correctly if it contains easily articulated sounds as in *bow, boat, ball, doll, home, mama, daddy, arm, mouth, thumb* and *fell.* In words like *car, coat,* and *book* the child may repeat only the vowels, since these are what he hears as *ar, oa,* and *oo.* These partial words should be accepted temporarily. As soon as the child learns to produce *k,* it should be incorporated into the word. Most normally hearing children correct their own speech errors over a period of years, but deaf children must be helped to do this, for they lack the power of self-correction. At this stage the teacher does not stop to correct every word a child says. She gladly accepts any oral communication the child offers. She constantly evaluates the child's imitative powers and, when she sees that he can perceive some of the details of speech production, she helps him toward correct articulation. The profoundly deaf child will have to depend on tactile as well as visual, kinesthetic and auditory sense impressions for gaining knowledge of speech production. He should have plenty of opportunity to feel the teacher's face when she and the child are conversing at close range. She may tell a story to one or two children while they stand close to her and feel her face when she talks. She should use a natural well pitched pleasantly modulated voice so that the pattern she furnishes will be a desirable one for the child to imitate. Should a deaf child use a shrill or loud strained voice during his spontaneous vocalizing, she should call his attention to the necessity for subduing it. She asks him to use his "pretty" voice. Such a child should have a great many chances to feel normal speech, so that when he comes to use his voice for speech it will fall within the range of normal production.

Five-year-olds are ready for learning. Their interests are expanding with a growing knowledge of their environment. Five-year-olds love to make things. They still need opportunities to experiment with materials and express themselves freely through art media.

Teachers should plan experiences for these children which reinforce the language emphasized in the past year and look forward to the language the children will need to express themselves more fully than they have previously.

Excursions into the neighborhood may be increased. A visit to a pet shop, the Humane Society's kennels, a trip to the store for ingredients for cup cakes, or for boxes or crates to build a house, a trip to see Santa at Christmas time, a trip to the barber shop for a haircut for one of the children, a trip to the drugstore for an ice cream treat—all serve to give the children experiences for a wider vocabulary and to establish that to which they have already been exposed. In kindergartens for hearing children excursions are taken to the airport, police station, post office, and the like. This kind of trip, while excellent for enlarging concepts of community life is still somewhat premature for five-year-old deaf children from the point of view of language development. While it is commendable that a child know and be able to say, "The policeman is my friend," such abstractions must be deferred. They should not be taught at the expense of the speech needs for everyday living.

Schoolroom experiences which serve the purposes outlined above include the building of a house of crates and boxes, playing house, dressing up in adult clothes, dressing and undressing dolls, washing and ironing doll clothes, washing doll dishes, having doll parties and playing doctor and nurse. Making airplanes of wood, building a schoolbus with blocks and going for make-believe rides can be used to foster the language the children need to express their needs and wants.

Hallowe'en with its pumpkin, Thanksgiving with its turkeys,

Christmas with its toys and Easter with its rabbit carry emotional association for the children rather than seasonal connotations. Not until children are about seven do they understand the passage of the seasons as such. Holidays should be celebrated but not emphasized. Five-year-olds do, however, gain clear concepts of *today, yesterday* and *tomorrow,* and begin to use the phrase *after a while* and *before.* Calendar work is still related to everyday happenings.

Number concepts begin to emerge at the five-year level. Children recognize groups of 2, 3, 4 and possibly 5 objects. They recognize that these quantities are made up of equal or unequal parts, as four has two equal parts of two. Rational counting begins at this level also. Any experiences which lend themselves to clarification of number concepts should be utilized. Children may count napkins, cups, spoons and cookies for a party and chairs for visitors.

Children at the five-year level should begin to appreciate that sentences are used to express thoughts. Though they still depend upon single words to communicate even complicated ideas or to ask questions, they must be led to using simple sentences themselves. These sentences must develop within the framework of the children's language understanding and speech capabilities. Many of these sentences will be learned as formulas suitable to certain occasions as: *Come, I forgot, I know, May I have some water? I love you.* Some will grow out of unusual situations as: *I fell, I coughed, We laughed.* Others may be related to a desire to display possessions as: *I have a doll, I have a book, I have a gun, I have a car.* All will have to be repeated countless times in the coming year before they become established as the children's own. Still others are inspired by planned experiences as: (at the park) *We saw a boat, We saw some ducks.*

Stories may also serve as the basis of language stimulation at this level. "The Three Bears," "Little Black Sambo" and "The Three Little Kittens" are easily dramatized. Children are expected, at this level, to be able to arrange the pictures of the story in sequence quite independently. They may act out the story as the teacher tells it. She may stop from time to time to ask the characters to speak appropriate lines. In the "Three Bears," Goldilocks may say of the three bowls of porridge as she tastes each one, "It is hot," "It is cold," "It is good"; and later of each bed, "It is hard," "It is soft," "It is fine."

Many five-year-olds respond very well to printed words. Charts describing experiences may be lettered by the teacher and illustrated by the children. The vocabulary and sentence patterns used are those entirely familiar to the children in lip reading. Children are able to point out the sentence spoken by the teacher, or match illustrations to the story. Incomplete sentences and expressions are avoided. A chart such as

> Look, look
> See the ball.
> A red ball
> Oh, oh, oh

serves no purpose for deaf children. This form of language appears in many pre-primers and may be suitable for children who hear and speak in this peculiar fashion, but not for children who are trying to learn a basic language pattern.

A sentence may be lettered on each day of the large calendar to record the main event of the day. A child may keep a record of his own news in his own notebook. He may illustrate, "I have new shoes," though the teacher does the lettering for him. Such reading activities lead to a better understanding of language, and prepare the child for spoken language.

Before any child can say a sentence he should have developed fairly good imitative powers related directly to movements of the articulators. He should have learned to use a pleasant voice with controlled pitch; to pronounce vowels and consonants clearly in syllables. He should have a rudimentary understanding of rhythm and a capacity to produce sentence-length breath.

It is apparent that if children with profound losses are to learn to talk they will need specific help in developing intelligible speech. While a great deal of their day will be devoted to free play and planned experiences informally carried out, special periods for speech help should be included in their programs. Most five-year-olds can attend to speech for a period of five or ten minutes. Several very short periods during a single day— two or three in a morning if the child attends school for half a

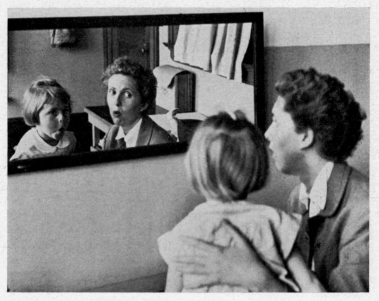

Visual clues along with kinesthetic and auditory clues are used to help the deaf child acquire speech and language.

day, and one or two in the afternoon—are needed to help develop speech skills. These lessons should be directly related to the child's language needs. If the child has attempted to say, "I have a book," and says "I uv a boo," the teacher's goals are as follow: addition of an aspiration before the *a* in "have," clearly articulated vowels, addition of a *k* to "book" and a rhythmic presentation of the sentence in one breath.

The Elementary School Years

During the years which children with severe and profound hearing losses spend in the elementary school they should be steadily gaining power in self-expression. Whereas the nursery school emphasized the receptive aspects of language acquisition, the emphasis in the elementary school is on guiding children into using correct language and intelligible speech.

Children in the primary grades (1 through 3) become very much interested in the external world and in the community. They are able to furnish some of their own discipline. Real friends begin to play an important role in their lives. The planned experiences for primary children will include many trips into the community. They will study its stores, its parks, its homes and its occupations. They learn about plants and growing things in gardens. They learn about the products of the farm. They discover through experiences both actual and vicarious, through movies and other visual means, the ways in which people travel from place to place. They learn about weather, temperature and the seasons. Their concepts of number relations are increasing. They learn the value of money, of units of measure and how to tell time. These experiences are the basis for language acquisition. Many new concepts have to be verbalized for the children in their spoken and written language. At this age deaf children begin to read books written for children who hear. It may require a year or two more for primary deaf children to progress commensurately with their hearing peers. But that is of little consequence if they really learn to use basic language forms correctly and automatically at this level. When children reach the intermediate and upper grades (4 through 8 or 9) their interests take them well beyond the confines of their homes and communities. They now become interested in faraway places and times past, in the how and why of natural phenomenon and in personal relations. They enjoy adventure, sports, excitement and tales of daring. Unless the children have acquired ability to handle basic language structures independently in the primary grades, they will be unprepared for the deluge which comes at the intermediate and upper grade levels. These children are called upon to absorb a great deal of subject matter through reading. The heavy vocabulary load associated with social studies, science, arithmetic, and the like, as well as the difficult sentence patterns and the complicated idioms required to express the more abstract concepts related to the subject matter is overwhelming indeed. The speed with which these materials are expected to be assimilated sometimes precludes sufficient drill in the speech and language aspects of the program. Parents often become concerned, as do teachers, at the slump into which many children seem to go in these grades. It is imperative that the vocabulary and language structures which are introduced at this level not only be clearly presented but well established in both the oral and written language of the children.

Language in the Elementary School

Language acquisition on the part of children demands that they gain control over the use of structures employed in language, and facility in the use of its vocabulary. Reading becomes an integral part of the language program at this level. All language lessons become reading lessons and all reading lessons must involve language learning. A summary of several studies relating to the language and reading abilities of the deaf will shed some light on the problems involved in the teaching of the language arts to children who have very limited hearing. Heider and Heider [16] compared the written compositions of deaf children between the ages of eleven and seventeen with those of hearing children between the ages of eight and fourteen. They found that the sentences of deaf children were shorter in number of words and number of clauses, and that the deaf used less complex sentences than hearing children. Upon analyzing the different forms of subordination, the reasons for the use of particular structures by the deaf were revealed. When word order of the subordinate clause differed from simple order as, subject, verb, object, when structure required organization of the whole sentence from the beginning, or when meaning was differentiated by a choice of connectives, the deaf avoided these structures.

Fusfeld [17] measured the academic achievement of 134 graduates of American residential schools who were applicants to the Preparatory Course of Gallaudet College using the Stanford Achievement Test, Advanced Battery, Form J, and found a median gross achievement of grade 9.2 with extremes falling in the latter half of the fourth grade and the first half of the twelfth. For the language test, consisting of a series of exercises requiring recognition of grammatic structure, capitalization and punctuation, the group median was grade 11.6, and for spelling it was 10.5. But in paragraph meaning the median was 8.2, and in word meaning 6.7. Applicants also wrote compositions on such subjects as "Advantages and Disadvantages of Deafness," "Science Is Rebuilding Our World" and "The Saturday Evening Post." "A tangled web type of language construction in which words occur in profusion but do not align themselves in orderly fashion" seemed characteristic of these written papers. Fusfeld concludes that the recognition of correct form does not insure grasping the sense of these forms in reading and produces very little skill in writing. He theorizes that the patternized type of language teaching which seems to be prevalent in schools for the deaf is responsible for this unfortunate state of affairs.

Pugh [18] studied the silent reading abilities of children in 56 schools for the deaf using the Iowa Silent Reading Test and the Durrell-Sullivan Reading Achievement Test. She found that some of the deaf children made maximum scores on the Iowa Test, equal to and exceeding the 99th percentile of hearing children who had been in school the same number of years, but that on all parts of the test the medians for children with hearing losses were lower than those for children who hear. The deaf showed greatest retardation in sentence meaning and in word meaning. They were more nearly like the hearing children on Alphabetizing and the Use of Index. The younger children showed less retardation than the older children, and though gradual progress was revealed for children who had attended school from 7 to 13 years, in some instances it was very slight. Pugh is careful to point out that there is no evidence to show that deaf children are inherently poor readers, since all deaf children are not retarded in reading. She suggests that improvement in reading must be based on developing special skills related to sentence meaning and word meaning, and to a general re-evaluation of methods of teaching reading to deaf children.

In practice it is not possible to separate the teaching of vocabulary from the teaching of sentence structures, or to divorce reading from language study. Only for purposes of the following discussion will they be considered individually.

The problem of teaching the structure of language artificially to children who have not been able to acquire language because they cannot hear has challenged educators since the first attempts were made to teach deaf children. Early efforts in the United States centered on the "grammatic" approach, as a result of the influence of the French teachers, de l'Epée, Sicard and Clerc. As children were admitted to school at ages 10, 11 or 12, they seemed likely victims for such practice. In the "grammatic" approach words were classified as to parts of speech and according to grammatic function. Rules of grammar served as the basis for the presentation of language and for the construction of sentences by the children. Meanings, as such, were largely ignored.

Not all American teachers were committed to the "grammatic" approach of teaching language to deaf children. From such distinguished 19th century European exponents of the oral method as Frederick Moritz Hill of Germany and Thomas Arnold of England came the precept that deaf children must be given the opportunity to learn language through immediate association with actual experiences related closely to their interests.[19] One of the first practitioners of this approach in the United States was David Greenberger, principal of the school now known as Lexington School for the Deaf, where his influence is still felt. Greenberger believed that deaf children should be given the opportunity to learn language to suit their needs at the time they felt the need. He eschewed any attempt to organize language presentation formally, but believed strongly in having children practice correct language in natural situations.[20] He believed with Arnold that words were not to be taught alone, but that thoughts were to be embodied in sentences. The early advocates of the education of the very young child, like Mary McCowan, realized that a grammatic approach to teaching language was entirely unsuitable for preschool children. The "natural" approach is based on the premise that language to be meaningful must be directly related to ideas and concepts derived from children's interests and experiences. The previous section on the nursery school described this approach without naming it.

Many schemes have been devised which were intended to visualize word relationships for the deaf child. One of these was contrived by Sicard in the late 18th century. In his system, numerals were placed over the components of a sentence as:

1	2	3	4	5
(subj.)	(verb)	(obj.)	(prep.)	(obj. of prep.)
Cows	eat	grass	in	summer.

This procedure was expected to help deaf children construct sentences correctly according to the prescribed grammatic rule.[20]

In the 1870's, Richard Storrs of the Hartford School used symbols together with "sentence maps" to clarify sentence and question forms. These symbols were used with memorized language. A few of the 47 symbols follow:

$\perp$ noun

$\perp'$ possessive case

$\checkmark$ verb

∞ conjunction

In a symbolized sentence as "The girl cried," person, number and tense were indicated. Grammar was supposedly expedited by the use of these symbols. The symbols were taught before the facts which illustrated them.[20]

While Storrs' symbols were not widely used because of their complexity and abstraction, those introduced by George Wing at the Minnesota School for the Deaf in the 1880's are still in use there and in a few other schools in the United States. His was also a grammatic approach, and the symbols were designed to explain the form, position and function of words within a sentence as:

posses-sive	subject	verb, past transitive	indirect object		adjec-tive	object	preposition-al phrase
1	*2*	✓	—o	3	3	o	————4
John's	mother	gave	him	a	new	football	for his birthday.

As soon as a child learned to write a sentence, the symbols were added to the written language. They were presented in conjunction with new language structures and were used in correcting children's language errors.

Just before 1900 the first book giving a definite plan for the development of language for beginners was published in America by Katherine Barry.[21] The "Five Slate System," as it is known, was really a revision of Sicard's system. Though "the idea before the word, the thought before the expression" was considered important, this system was based on grammatic principles. The analysis of sentences was done on a large set of slates reserved for the purpose. Children also had small slates of their own ruled into five columns. The first column was devoted to the subject of the verb, the second to the verb and its complement, the third to the object of the verb, the fourth to the preposition and the fifth to the object of the preposition. Pupils were made to analyze practically every sentence written by putting the person and things written about them in their respective places on the slates (see figure 3).

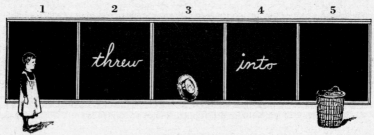

FIG. 3.—The Five Slate System.

Actually, a sixth column, "when," was later added to indicate time of action. Miss Barry outlined a definite order of presenting the grammatic principles from the simple to the more complex. Her system is still used in some American schools.

The most widely used device for teaching language today is the one introduced by Edith Fitzgerald in 1926. It is generally referred to as the Fitzgerald Key.[22] It is used wholly or in part in two-thirds of 132 schools for the deaf reporting in a survey of language methods in use in North America.[20] The Key is a synthesis of many approaches to language teaching, but with some original features. Like Barry's system, it makes use of columns, but in the Key appropriate headings are used to indicate the most common word order in English (see table 2). It also incorporates the use of a few symbols to indicate parts of speech as,

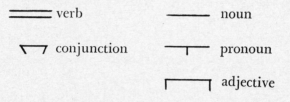

The Key was designed to aid in the systematic presentation of language to deaf children, within the framework of their needs and experiences. A sequence of presentation of language structures is indicated, though no specific order is prescribed.

Before the Key itself is used, children classify the words they have acquired through vocabulary study under such headings as *Who, What, How Many, Where.* These headings are known as "key words." Adjectives and verbs are grouped under their respective symbols. The Key is developed with the children as new language principles are introduced.* Eventually the order

---

* Language principles may be thought of as broadly encompassing: (1) the patterns of statements and questions as, *Subject, Verb, Object; Who* ——? (2) arrangements of words expressing relationships of grammatic structure as, *on the table,* (3) modifying elements as, *the big bad wolf;* He went *down quietly,* (4) verb tenses and verbal forms as, the past perfect tense and all its forms; infinitives, gerunds, participles, (5) the variants and inflected forms of adjectives and nouns as, *big, bigger, biggest; goose, geese; man's, men's,* (6) such grammatic items as indicate the presence or absence of a negative as, I haven't *any,* (7) items substituting for nouns as, *he, each, anybody.*

Table 2.—*The Fitzgerald Key with Illustrations of Sentences Written in the Key*

Subject	Verb	Ind.	Dir.	Adverbial Modifiers of Main Verb		
WHAT: WHO:	Pred. Adj. Pred. Noun Pred. Pron.	Obj.	Obj.	WHERE:	FOR—; HOW FAR: FROM—; HOW OFTEN: WITH—; HOW LONG: HOW: HOW MUCH: WHY: (IF)	WHEN:
		WHAT: WHOM: ( ) WHOM: WHAT:				
Father	bought	me a box of candy			for my birthday.	
I	know	that you have a dog at home.				
Jerry	likes	to play with his dog.				
We	will go		to Chicago	on the train		this summer.

284

of the elements of the sentence and the relationships of the modifying elements to the words they modify are learned through the use of this visual aid. Suggestions for building the Key are made in Fitzgerald's book. The Key serves as the basis for the understanding of question forms through its classification system. It serves as a self-correction device for children as they go about using new language forms.

It is quite important when employing any device in language instruction that the means do not become the end, or that the crutch which the device may become does not interfere with the children's ability to move ahead freely, steadily and independently. Successful teaching of the structures of English demands that:

1. the most important items of language be selected, arranged and taught in a properly related sequence, suitable to the age and background of the children.

2. these items be presented in relation to the experiences and interests of the children.

3. there be constant clarification of the language being taught.

4. children be given sufficient opportunity to practice using the language presented so that it can be stabilized. This requires that the children, not the teacher, do most of the talking as well as most of the writing.

5. there be constant review of all the language the children have learned in the past.

6. there be adequate opportunity for recognition and preparation for new language forms to be taught in the future.

The teacher may refer to publications by Buell,[23] Croker, Jones and Pratt,[24] Fitzgerald,[22] Pugh [25] and to the Central Institute Outline [26] for the orderly presentation of language principles.

A general scheme for the presentation of language principles follows:

I. *Preparation.* The teacher uses the language principle well in advance in many actual situations in lip reading and in writing.

II. *Introduction for Study by Children.* The teacher introduces the language principle in an actual situation requiring the use of the specific principle.

III. *Planned Repetition for Reinforcement and Clarification of the Pattern.* The teacher sets up situations in the form of games, or through use of visual aids which elicit the desired language pattern. The pattern may be further clarified at this time and the limits of its use set.

IV. *Incidental Use by Children With Help of Teacher.* As the occasion demands, children are held to the use of the principle. If the child has difficulty in recalling the principle, further drill may be necessary until pattern is more firmly established.

V. *Automatic and Habitual Use of Principle by Children.* The children have mastered the principle when they use it spontaneously and correctly at the proper time without help from the teacher.

The following lesson plan illustrates how these stages can be applied to the teaching of a language principle to seven-year-olds.

THE LANGUAGE PRINCIPLE: "WHERE IS ——?"

I. Preparation	T.*	Where is your handkerchief, John?
	C.	In my pocket.
teacher uses	T.	Wipe your face, please.
principle		
well in ad-	T.	Where is your eraser, Bill?
vance in	C.	In my desk.
many actual	T.	Please give it to me.
situations	T.	Where is your scarf, Linda?
in lip	C.	I don't know.
reading and	T.	Find it and put it on before you go out to play.
in writing		
	T.	Where is David this morning?
	C.	He is at home. He is sick.
	T.	Where is your hearing aid, Sally?
	C.	At home.

* *T* stands for *Teacher,* and *C* for *Child.*

II. Introduction for Study

teacher introduces principle in an actual situation

One day the children come to school and see on the blackboard:

Where is ——?

During a recess period the teacher has removed the very conspicuous Valentine box from the table and placed it in her cupboard away from sight because the children seem to have been too distracted by its presence. When the children return from recess, they say excitedly:

"Box? Where?"

The teacher then writes on the blackboard,

Where is the Valentine box?

and asks each child to repeat the question. The children are able to do so because all the words in the sentence are familiar to them, though not in this particular sequence. If they were not, this particular combination would not have been chosen to introduce the question form.

The teacher then explains that the Valentine box is in the cupboard and will remain there until the afternoon Valentine party. The question form is then recorded on a chart with other question forms that the children use.

Who?
What did —— do?
May I have —— ?
Where is —— ?

III. Planned Repetition for re-enforcement and clarification of pattern

teacher sets up situations

(1) The teacher has hidden various objects which the children are in the habit of taking outdoors with them at recess time—football, dodge ball, jump rope. The teacher asks a child to get the jump rope. Child goes to the usual place but can't see it.

T. I will tell you where the jump rope is if you ask me a question.

Child cannot remember the pattern, so the teacher asks child to refer to the chart. Child does not yet recognize the form to be used, so teacher writes on the blackboard:

Where is —— ?

which will elicit the desired language. The principle may be further clarified at this time and the limits of its use set

The child looks at the pattern, turns toward the teacher and says

C. Where is the jump rope?
T. It is behind the piano, I think.

Child goes for the jump rope.
The same procedure is used to locate the dodge ball and the football.

(2) Children cover their eyes while teacher takes one of a group of six or seven objects from the table in front of the class and places it somewhere behind the children. Children have to determine which object has been removed in order to ask the question.

C. Where is the hammer?
T. In my desk drawer. It is in my desk drawer.

Child gets hammer and replaces it among the objects on the table. Child then becomes teacher and hides another object.

C2. Where is the red pencil?
C1. Under John's desk. The pencil is under John's desk.

Child gets pencil and returns it to the teacher. Second child then becomes teacher. This procedure is followed so that each child has an opportunity to hide an object and ask a question.

(3) One child hides while a second child closes his eyes. On signal the latter asks any one of the other children:

C1. Where is Linda?
C2. In the coat room.

Child finds Linda and another proceeds to hide and ask a question.

(4) So that children do not get the idea that they must be blindfolded to ask a question, the following game does not use a blindfold.

The teacher has placed various objects in unusual places about the room without the children's being aware of it.

T. My purse is not in my cupboard. You don't know where my purse is. Ask me where my purse is.
C1. Where is your purse?
T. In my desk.

Child retrieves purse and teacher asks child to put it in her cupboard.

T. You don't know where Bill's cap is.
C2. Where is my cap?
T. In your desk. Please hang it up now.

T. You don't know where Sally's pencil is.
C3. Where is Sally's pencil?
T. In my pocket.

All children have an opportunity to ask questions upon suggestions offered by the teacher.

IV. Incidental Use by Children with Help of Teacher

A child needs some paste but cannot locate the jar. He comes to the teacher and says, "Paste," pointing to where it should be.

T. Please ask me a question and I will tell you where the paste is.

as the occasion demands the children are held to use of principle

The child still seems confused so the teacher refers the child to the chart containing the question forms. He recognizes the correct question form.

C. Where is the paste?

if clarification is necessary the

T. It is in Miss Brown's room. You may go to Miss Brown's room and get the paste. What will you say?
C. Where is the paste?

principle has   **T.** No, you know where the paste is. It is in Miss
not been   Brown's room. Ask Miss Brown if you may have the
well enough   paste. What will you say?
established   **C.** May I have the paste, please?
and more   **T.** That's right. Run along.
drill is
necessary

V. Automatic   **C1.** Where is Sally?
and Habitual   **T.** She went to the office.
Use of
Principle   **C2.** Where is my space helmet?
by Children   **T.** I put it in my cupboard.

                C3. Where is the moth?
                T. It flew away while you were at lunch.

Vocabulary in the Elementary School

Helping children acquire an adequate vocabulary is one of the major tasks of the teacher. The studies by Pugh [18] and Fusfeld [17] indicate that, in general, understanding and use of vocabulary by deaf children is quite deficient. The deaf child is required to learn countless numbers of words as they appear in basic English constructions, in idiomatic expressions and in figures of speech. The fact that most words have multiple meanings considerably complicates vocabulary study. It has been estimated that a child will have to add at least five new words to his vocabulary every day in the primary grades and from seven to nine in the intermediate grades in order to enable him to read in books. Thus, in a short time a child is expected to accumulate a vocabulary of thousands of words as one might accumulate buttons in a large box. Utter confusion may be the result unless some orderly arrangement or organization is devised to expedite their use. The collector may sort his buttons in various ways according to size, shape, color or kind of material, or according to both color and size or shape and size, as desired. They may be placed in smaller boxes within the larger box, or in envelopes within the smaller boxes, and rearranged any time to suit the requirements of the occasion. Unless a person looks over his collection from time to time, he may easily forget what is in it. Just so, there must be organization of vocabulary and constant reorganization to keep the items freshly in mind, the new words always related to some category of known words or ideas. Vocabulary can be remembered and used only if sufficient provision is made for its recall and use. It has been stated that though some words can be learned and remembered with only one contact, it takes about sixty contacts generally for a word to be incorporated into a deaf child's vocabulary.[27]

Vocabulary study begins with the naming of visible objects, actions and demonstrable qualities. Later children must learn words of various degrees of abstraction. They will have to make generalizations such as the one that *barns, schools, garages, sheds, apartment houses* and the like are *buildings*. Abstractions on a higher level, as *honesty, mistreatment* and *extravagance* will have to be related not only to other words but to the larger ideas from which the abstractions have been derived. If children are to gain clear concepts of what words mean and how they are used, they must be presented within the context of a sentence, for the only true meaning of a word is derived from the situation in which it is used.[28] Dictionary definitions are not helpful if usage is the objective.

The organization of vocabulary will depend on the interests and needs of the children and on the curriculum which is being followed. Every day incidental opportunities will present themselves for the introduction of new vocabulary. These situations should be capitalized on during the entire school life of deaf children. If, in the primary grades, a class is studying about stores in the neighborhood, means of transportation or the products of the farm, vocabulary will be developed around these subjects. It will be largely descriptive and objective rather than abstract. For this reason pictures may be used to good advantage. Concepts should be strengthened through use of pictures, and not introduced by them.

The descriptive vocabulary of the primary grades becomes the basis for the more abstract vocabulary used in the intermediate and upper grades when the children study the occupations of certain geographic regions, the transportation and distribution of goods in remote parts of the world and the importance of farm products in the economy of the country. The preparation of vocabulary for the study of specific subject matter must be gradual but definitely planned over a period of many years. For instance, if children are to understand the abstract vocabulary related to democratic government and politics, it is necessary and desirable to set up a democratic classroom situation even for young children. There may be a class "leader" who is responsible for certain duties as taking attendance and collecting lunch money. This child may be *elected,* the children *voting* each week for a new leader. If there is a school *council,* the elected *representatives* may become one of its *members.* Here some *rules* or *laws* of school conduct may be *formulated, discussed* and *passed. Monitors* or school safety *guards* may help *enforce* the rules. By the time children are expected to understand the complications of city, state and national governments, the understandings as well as the vocabulary which they have gained through real experience will be valuable indeed.

The vocabulary of specific subject matter may often be developed through daily experiences before it is encountered more or less formally in reading materials. For instance, during a spectacularly heavy rain storm the class discussion might center on the *downpour,* and from it would grow an extensive vocabulary related to rain. Children would list the kinds of rain as, *a drizzle, a mist, a shower, a thunderstorm;* they would describe how the rain comes down when it is *light,* when it is *heavy.* As the sidewalks dry, a discussion of *vapor, evaporation* and *cloud formation* could result. When children eventually come to study the climates of various regions of the earth, the vocabulary they have learned will serve as a basis for the deeper study of weather and climate.

If children in the upper grades are faced with having to learn fifty or a hundred new words every day or two, in order to read a certain required section of a book on a certain subject, the task becomes insurmountable. To avoid such an impasse a long range program for the development of vocabulary related to special school subjects becomes mandatory.

Besides organizing vocabulary around incidental daily happenings, events or news, around planned activities or units and around the subject matter fields as arithmetic, social studies and science, it is necessary to make provision for a program of word study based on the expansion of the basic vocabulary which the children learn during the first four or five years in school. Such study is intended to fill in any gaps left by the other approaches. A special period of the day should be devoted to it in the late primary, the intermediate and upper grades. The new words a child learns should always be associated with the old, thereby reviewing them and relating the new to the known.

For example, the noun *coat* becomes familiar to most deaf children at an early age. Later the child learns the parts of the coat as, *sleeves, pockets, buttons, collar, zipper* and *lining.* He may also learn the names of other outer garments as, *raincoat, stormcoat, overcoat, jacket, shortie* and *blazer,* so that he can speak more precisely about these articles. Eventually he will learn to identify a particular coat as a *fur coat,* an *orlon coat,* a *wool coat,* or a *beautiful coat,* a *warm coat,* a *shabby coat* or an *expensive coat.* He will learn that he can *put on* a coat, *take off* a coat, *button* a coat, *pick up* a coat, *drag* a coat, *tear* a coat, *lose* a coat and *press* a coat. He learns that a coat can *blow open, shrink* and *wear out.*

During the first years a child is in school he learns to say *I ran,* since he engages freely in this activity. Soon he observes that animals run, and eventually learns that even *water,* a *train,* a *motor* and *one's nose* can run. Much later he will be called on to understand and interpret expressions like these: *The idea ran through his head,* or *He ran the race of life successfully,* as well as other abstractions and idioms connected with this very versatile word. In the meantime he also discovers that a person who runs quickly for a short distance *dashes,* and one who runs exceptionally fast *streaks.* All the synonyms and derivatives as well as all the meanings of the basic verbs should be organized for him in some fashion so as to make meaning clear, and recall instantaneous. His knowledge of a particular word will be gained over a period of years, but his access to this knowledge must be a ready one.

As for adjectives, a child early learns the word *small*. He learns that a chair, a doll or a piece of cake can be small. This is a relative concept and more difficult to make clear to a little child. He also learns that *big* is the opposite of *small*. Later, he learns the synonyms of these words: *tiny, wee, minute; large, enormous, huge.* He can compare them not only as opposites but can arrange them in order according to size: *minute, tiny, small; big, huge, enormous.* He learns that he can say a *wee fairy* but not a *wee chair;* an *enormous meal* but seldom an *enormous woman.* Each and every word in the child's early vocabulary should serve as a basis for expansion of his vocabulary in his later school life.

Word study of this kind may be organized around large categories of words as *movements, communication, sounds, sensations* and *intellectual faculties.* It is necessary of course to make many subgroupings within the large categories. Children may learn how people move; how animals move; how water moves; how trains, boats, and airplanes move; and how clouds move. In relation to the category of *communication,* children might study units based on sounds that animals make, how people communicate without using speech and how they communicate by using speech. Each unit would again be subdivided for purposes of study. For example the basic word *say* may be used as the foundation for study of hundreds of related words which in themselves are organized some way within the unit on "how people speak": as synonyms, *spoke, talked, told, uttered;* according to degree of loudness, *whispered, muttered, mumbled, shouted;* according to intersocial affection, *persuaded, advised, convinced, implored, threatened, argued;* imparting news, *reported, rumored, gossiped, tattled, informed, broadcast;* according to derivation, *argued—argument, threatened—threat, reported—report, advised—advice.* A study of prefixes and suffixes serves as a further basis of organization and reorganization of vocabulary. Idioms are to be treated just as any other vocabulary item. They should be related to known words and should be organized within various units according to meaning. It is necessary to recall and use them frequently if they are to be understood by the children.

A record should be kept with the child of all the words and idioms he learns. A large looseleaf notebook seems most suitable for the child's ready use. It can, and should be referred to time and time again. It should not contain a helter-skelter list of words, but it should be organized according to the categories of words being studied. Words should always be recorded in context and, if possible, illustrated with pictures. Wall charts containing new words may be displayed and picture files of words suitably organized as reference materials may be provided for the children.

The alert teacher will encourage and guide the child in using his new vocabulary in every possible situation: when he reports on his daily activities, during class discussions, when he writes letters and in his original compositions. Many good suggestions for vocabulary development may be found in current periodicals. The teacher is urged to refer to them.[29-32] A thesaurus is an invaluable aid in preparing vocabulary units.

A lesson plan for teaching vocabulary related to the word "argue" follows. This plan was used with a class of children in the upper grades.

I. Introduction *the teacher creates a setting for the new word if it has not arisen spontaneously*	The teacher dramatizes what would happen in a situation in which two cars collide. She has two toy cars and names the driver of each car, though she impersonates each of the drivers. The men begin talking quietly at first and then, as it turns out that each thinks he is right, they both become angry.
II. Presentation	*T.* The two men *spoke angrily to each other* about the accident. Who can write that sentence on the blackboard?

*(a) teacher
tries to
elicit the
word from
the children
as she relates
it to known
vocabulary*

*(b) the word is
presented
orally
first
and then
in writing*

(Child writes sentence. Teacher underlines "spoke angrily to each other.")

T. Does anyone know another way to say this?
C. The two men *talked* angrily to each other about the accident.
T. Yes, that is correct, but I will tell you still another way to say it: "The two men *argued* about the accident." Will each of you say the new word for me, "argued."

(Each child says the word and is corrected if he makes an error.)

T. Will someone try to write the word right here, below "spoke angrily to each other."

(A child attempts to write it and is helped with the spelling.)

——argued——

*III. Clarifica-
tion of use
of word*

T. Can any of you think of a time when you argued about something?
Beth. I argued my sister about my swimming suit.

*(a) the limits
in which
the word
can be used
are defined*

From the children's contributions, the following sentences evolved after much discussion, correction and clarification of the use of the word in a sentence.

Beth and her sister argued about her swimming suit.
Beth argued with her sister about her swimming suit.
Beth argued with her sister about who would wear the swiming suit.

The pitcher and the umpire argued with each other.
The pitcher argued with the umpire about a called strike.
The pitcher argued with the umpire over a strike which he had called.

*(b) the
meanings of
the word are
enlarged to
fit the needs
of the class*

T. Sometimes people argue when they are angry, but there are times when they argue for the enjoyment of it. They may not agree, but they compare their ideas in a friendly fashion. Two men were talking about last week's election. They did not agree, but they did not grow angry. They had a friendly

*(c) attention
is called
to words
with same
derivation*

*IV. Relation
to former
vocabulary*

*(a) teacher
recalls with
children some
other situa-
tions
which can be
related to
use of new
verb*

*(b) vocabulary
is organized
according
to some
scheme in
relation to
other known
words*

argument. Argue and *argument* are two good words to remember. *Argue* is a verb, and *argument,* a noun.

Can someone tell me about Beth and her sister, using the word *argument?*

Sally. Beth had an argument with her sister about her swimming suit.

T. Good. Was it a friendly argument, Beth?

Beth. No, I was angry for a little while.

T. Perhaps you *lost your head* for a minute, Beth. Do you think the baseball pitcher *lost his head?*

John. Yes, I think he lost his head.

T. That's right, we can say that. Can anyone remember another way to express that idea?

Fred. The pitcher *lost his temper.*

Jerry. The pitcher *did not control his temper.*

T. Very good. Now let us see if we can recall some of the other words we have been studying. You remember, we talked about the words *quarreled, disagreed* and *agreed* yesterday. Which words express unfriendly feelings and which friendly feelings? Let us write them here in these two columns. Who wants to be first?

(Children volunteer and the following statements are written on the board first, and then recorded in notebooks.)

Unfriendly feelings

1. (Someone) disagreed with (someone) about (something).
2. (Someone) quarreled with (someone) over (something).
3. (Someone) argued with (someone) about (something).
4. (Someone) argued with (someone) over (something).

Friendly feelings

1. (Someone) agreed with (someone) about (something).
2. (Someone) consented to (something).
3. (Someone) had a friendly argument with (someone).
4. (Someone) recommended (something) to (someone).
   (Someone) recommended (someone) to (someone).

*V. Review
and Drill*

Draw a Circle Around the Correct Word

*review may
be oral or
written*

1. People often "lose their heads" when they: agree with someone, argue about something, consent to something.

*multiple
choice is used
as an exercise
of recognition
rather than
as a test*

2. Two women were discussing a book. They both said they liked it very much. They: disagreed about the book, argued about it, agreed about it.

3. A man and his friend enjoyed discussing politics. They had conflicting opinions about a new tax. They: had a friendly argument about the new tax, quarreled about it, agreed about it.

4. A girl wished to visit her cousin in Chicago. She asked her mother if she could go. Her mother said she could. Her mother: consented to letting her go, recommended that she should go, argued over her going.

*VI. Test
frequently*

Write a sentence about each of the incidents below using a word we have been studying.

1. Two little boys were talking about their fathers. One little boy said his father was very strong. The other said his father was stronger because he could lift a row boat. The other boy said his father was stronger because he could push his car. They began to talk very fast and they grew just a little angry as they talked about whose father was stronger.

2. John and Bill were playing catch. Bill threw the ball through a neighbor's window. He said to John, "You should have caught the ball." John said, "You threw it too high." Bill said, "You weren't looking." The boys became very angry as they talked about whose fault it was that the window was broken.

3. Mrs. Jones and Mrs. Smith were talking about the weather. Mrs. Smith said she liked warm weather and Mrs. Jones said she did, too.

Reading in the Elementary School

A large body of literature dealing with developmental and remedial reading for hearing children has accumulated in recent years. A perusal of this literature brings out two clear facts: one, that learning to read is a very complex process and, two, that many children in the ordinary school do not learn to read efficiently despite the fact that they come into the elementary school with several thousand words in their vocabularies and a knowledge of spoken language. Their first task is to learn to recognize and identify printed symbols and associate them with the language they already know. Is it any wonder, then, that deaf children who enter the elementary school from nursery school with only one or two, or at most several hundred words in their vocabularies and very little concrete knowledge of the use of connected language, find it difficult to learn to read at all?

Reading must be viewed as a language activity rather than as a school subject.[18, 33] As a process it involves thinking, since thoughts are expressed largely by words. As children gain in ability to use words precisely for exact shades of meaning, thinking becomes increasingly verbal. In order to read with comprehension children must know the meanings of the words and understand the language patterns represented by the printed text. Children who acquire skill in speaking and writing are better able to dig out the meanings in difficult reading materials. Without language proficiency, no matter how well children can perceive, recognize, identify or pronounce a printed word, the content of reading material will be unintelligible to them.[15] Thus, the capacity of deaf children to understand and use language cannot be overemphasized as a concomitant of the reading program.

Let us consider the importance of reading to children with severe and profound hearing losses. The printed or written form of language tends to strengthen and clarify the spoken form which is often vague and ambiguous on the lips.[4] Reading becomes an important tool for these children as they grow older and are expected to add to their store of knowledge through reading. Those children who learn to enjoy reading will find it a rewarding lifetime activity.

Though six and a half years is the age generally recommended for beginning reading with children who hear, a deaf child who attends nursery school will have been introduced to the printed symbol at a time when the teacher believes that his emotional maturity, his visual perceptual maturity and his intelligence warrant it. This is done to give the child a more complete impression of language than can be derived from that perceived fragmentarily on the lips and only partially through the ear.

In the nursery school, as well as in the first year in elementary school while the child is adding to his knowledge of words and language through lip reading and through his ear, the teacher can explore his visual skills. The teacher should try to discover if the child is able to make gross visual discriminations, like noticing the difference between a picture of a box and that of a ball, seeing likenesses and differences among a series of items, observing sizes and shapes, observing position or place and observing internal details in pictures. She should explore his ability to recognize parts of things that belong together and his ability to generalize by grouping items such as toys into their proper categories. The child should have an opportunity to hear stories, to dramatize stories and to arrange picture stories in a sequential order. Through the use of pictures his ability to see causal relationships can also be explored.[15] Through exercises in which he matches object with object, picture with object, printed form with object and printed form with picture, he eventually learns to recognize and identify the printed word as having symbolic meaning.[14] These exercises are not presented to force reading, and no effort is made at this stage to have him vocalize what he reads.

The elementary school program is at first merely an extension of the program of the earlier years. All the language the children learn through their activities and experiences is presented orally and then in print in the form of flash cards, or material typed on large primer typewriters for the child's personal books. The language used consists of the basic structures which the children are learning.

The first reading charts are simple ones, consisting perhaps of a single verb used with a single noun. They grow more complex as the children's understanding of language is developed (see table 3).

TABLE 3.—*Examples of Charts for Children Entering Elementary School Years*

I	II	III
Hats John made a hat. Linda made a hat. Bob made a hat. Sue made a hat. Jill made a hat. Nicky made a hat.	We made cookies. We ate the cookies. We made cocoa. We drank the cocoa.	*Cup Cakes* We went to the store. We bought some cake-mix. We made cup cakes. We will have a party.
Our Toys Jill has a doll. Sue has a yo-yo. Nicky has a gun. Bob has a car. Linda has a ball. John has a truck.	Jill has a new car. The car is red. Linda has a ball. The ball is big.	*Bob's Dog* Bob has a dog. He can stand up. He can roll over. He can shake hands. He is a smart dog.
Outdoor Fun Sue ran. Nicky ran. Bob ran. Linda ran. John ran. Jill ran.	Bob ran. He fell. Sue ran. She did not fall.	*Tag* John and Nicky played tag. John ran. Nicky ran. They ran and ran.

After children have read dozens of experience charts, imaginary stories using the familiar experiences and language can be introduced. The children first dramatize them as a check on comprehension, and then illustrate them. The stories may be gathered into book form, a large sized book for class use, and typed and duplicated copies for the children's own books. The first "story" might require that only one actor perform one action:

| A boy ran. | A girl fell. | A boy threw a ball. | A dog ran. |

Then "stories" requiring two actions and/or two actors can be introduced:

| A boy ran and fell. |

A girl had a doll.

She kissed the doll.

A boy threw a ball.

A girl caught the ball.

A girl had some gum.

She chewed the gum.

A boy had a dog.

The boy gave the dog a bone.

Dean fell.

He hurt his knee.

He did not cry.

Charts requiring greater imagination may be presented next. The children have to read something into these situations in order to dramatize them.

A boy had a penny.

He went to the store.

He bought some gum.

A girl's mother gave her a book.

The girl sat down and read the book.

Children enjoy riddle charts.

I am red.

I grow on a tree.

What am I?

I am small.

I am black.

I say meow, meow.

What am I?

In "What happened?" charts the children finish the "stories."

Bob and his dog went out doors. _____.

Sue dropped her doll. The doll broke. _____.

These charts or typed paragraphs are read silently, but if a child does read orally, the exercise may be considered a speech lesson, rather than a reading lesson.

Teachers must exercise considerable skill in constructing charts, making sufficient provision for repetition of new vocabulary, and writing in clearly unified paragraphs, keeping phrases together and spacing sentences properly. Charts for primary children should consist of from three to eight sentences in one or two paragraphs. For children in the intermediate grades, several paragraphs are suitable.

Eventually the time will come when the teacher will wish to introduce the children to book reading. She has at her disposal a vast amount of attractive material in the form of basic readers, social science textbooks, science texts, story books, juvenile classics and literature. All of these books have been written for children who hear, and since there are no books written especially for children with hearing losses, the teacher must make her selection from among those available. Undoubtedly she will choose books belonging to a series of basic readers for use in the developmental reading program. These readers generally reflect the experiences and interests of middle class American children. Vocabulary is controlled carefully, at least through the third grade level. Since books are written with the assumption that even beginners will be familiar with the many uses of words and will be able to use simple, compound and complex sentences, the structures appearing in the simplest readers at the lowest levels are very complicated. All the verb tenses and verbal forms—infinitives, participles and gerunds—are used in books beyond the primer level. Inverted sentence order appears even in primers, and idioms occur in great profusion from the fourth grade on. If a semantic count is made of the vocabulary items in any book, the number of words listed as new in the rear of the book could easily be increased by 30 per cent.

The teacher's task is to select reading material suitable to the interests and language abilities of each child. She will have to familiarize herself with the contents of a great many books before she decides on the level of the books she will use. Her judgment will be based largely on the informal evaluation of the child's abilities, rather than on formal tests, since scores on standardized tests do not necessarily reflect a deaf child's real capacity to read. If a deaf child is confronted with too difficult material, he will either become so discouraged as to reject reading entirely, or will go through the motions of reading to please the teacher, looking for a familiar word here and there, skipping over unknown portions and comprehending little or nothing of the printed text. In either case the objectives of a good reading program are defeated.

In order to stimulate a child's abiding interest in reading, and to lead him to independence in reading, the program will have to be very carefully planned. First, the teacher will have to be sure that the child has had experiences, either actual or vicarious, similar to those discussed in the book. Then she will have to prepare *well in advance* the difficult and strange concepts appearing within the book, the new vocabulary, idioms, and strange sentence structures. Above all she will have to give daily guidance and direction in the reading of the individual selections.

When children are ready to read in books, it is important that they begin to learn the vocabulary related to the book and its parts, and to the act of reading. A lesson is expedited if children can respond to directions given orally as "Open your books to page ___," "Look at the picture on page sixteen." All the words related to parts of the book are taught when needed: *front cover, back cover, the title, the author, the top of the page, the bottom of the page, table of contents, illustrations, glossary, index, publisher,* as well as the contents of the book: *a word, a sentence, the last sentence, the first line, a statement, a ques-*

tion, a paragraph, the first paragraph, a story, a humorous story, a hero tale, a joke, a riddle, a conversation, a description, and finally, the verbs that are used during a lesson: *read, read to yourself, tell, tell about, turn to page ___, find the word that tells ___.*

If a teacher selects a pre-primer as the first book that a child will read, she will find it nicely illustrated, but written in a style quite different from the basic structures she has been teaching her class. For example, *Look, look. Here I come. See, see. See what I have,* is a far cry from *I have a new doll* or *We went to the park.* The text makes about as much sense when read from the back to the front as from the front to the back of the book. The pictures alone carry the story along.

The teacher, then, has the choice of avoiding the pre-primer altogether, teaching the sentence forms used in the book as supplementary to the basic structures she has been teaching, or of discarding the printed text and substituting her own, written in language familiar to the children, and suited to the illustrations. Not all story units in pre-primers will lend themselves to this kind of revision, but selected ones, related to the children's experience can be utilized very satisfactorily in this way. Children are happy to read familiar material; parents are satisfied because the children are reading books; the teacher is satisfied because she knows the children understand what they read.

There are many approaches to organizing the reading program. If a school system requires that deaf children read a basic series from beginning to end, it is possible that a class may be reading Hallowe'en stories at Christmas time, and stories about a snowman in the spring time. The reading series can become a large factor in determining the curriculum, for in order to give children sufficient background and preparation for the stories in the reader, units of study will have to be based on them. All the arguments for reading straight through a basic series are found in published materials.[34] While this procedure may be very desirable for children who hear, it may not be entirely suitable for deaf children.

In some school systems a basic reading series is adopted, but

several supplementary books from other series are used at each
level of difficulty before proceeding to the next higher level in
the basic series. Though there is some correlation between vocabulary in the various series, it cannot be assumed that there
will be any degree of overlap of vocabulary items among them.
This type of organization requires careful preparation for every
book used.

If the curriculum of the school is based mainly on children's
needs and interests, the units of study decided upon for a certain
class may not coincide with the stories in a particular set of
readers. Under these circumstances the solution to the reading
problem is found in an integrated language-reading approach.
For example, a teacher who used this method selected a unit on
Transportation for a class of eight-year-olds who had been in
school for five years. She gathered in advance reading materials
from all possible sources: basic readers, social science texts, correlated film-texts [35] and story books. The children had actual
experiences riding on buses, trains and boats, and they saw
movies about these means of transportation. As the children
gained new concepts, these were verbalized and recorded in
chart form. But not only did the real and vicarious experiences
determine what language structures and vocabulary were to be
used in the unit, but the idioms, vocabulary and structures in
the reading material were anticipated and included in the language study. Each child read on his own level a great deal of
material related to the subject. In this integrated approach a
teacher has the advantage of making a wide choice of suitable
reading material, but also has the responsibility of seeing that
the children grow steadily in ability to read independently as
they progress through a series of units during the school year.

A program that concentrates only on the reading of subject
matter—as the social sciences or science—is certainly not a complete one. Children must not be denied the opportunity of reading fairy stories, humorous stories and adventure stories. The
common fairy tales should be familiar to the children before
they read them, just as hearing children are familiar with them
before they meet them in print. Storytelling should serve as an

interest-arousing device all during the elementary grades. The vocabulary of fairy stories and adventure stories is built up through storytelling and dramatization in advance of the reading.

Library periods can also be utilized to stimulate interest in reading. Deaf children, especially the younger ones, should not be turned loose in a library without some guidance, for they are not always capable of making good choices independently. A limited number of books may be displayed attractively on a reading table. From the display the children can choose the books they wish to take home. The books which children read for pleasure should be one grade level below those used in the developmental reading program.[36] Children are usually eager to tell about what they have read and should be given an opportunity to make some report, informal though it may be, on every book they read, thus providing the teacher with another check on their comprehension. A record of all the books the children read may be posted on the bulletin board. This, in turn, stimulates further reading.

Among some of the abilities that deaf children must develop if they are to become independent readers are:

1. Ability to recognize familiar words and language in print quickly.

2. Ability to attack words independently through phonetic clues, structural clues, context clues, and through use of the dictionary. (In many American schools for the deaf the scheme used to teach phonics is the one devised at Clarke School for the Deaf.[37] The Northampton Charts, containing the most ordinary spellings of our very unphonetic language, are introduced and built with each child as he acquires ability to use a particular sound or group of sounds in speech [see table 4]. A child who can identify, recognize and write the multiple spellings for the various English phonemes not only has at his fingertips a valuable aid for self-help in speech, but has a good basis for a more detailed study of phonics as related to reading. A summary of word identification skills to be developed is shown in table 5.)

TABLE 4.—*The Northampton Charts (Reproduced with permission of Clarke School for the Deaf, Northampton, Massachusetts)*

Consonant Sounds

h—				
wh	w—			
p	b	m		
t	d [1]	n	J	r—
k	g	ng		
c		n(k)		
ck				
f	v			
ph				
[1] th	[2] th			
[1] s	z			
c(e)	[2] s			
c(i)				
c(y)				
sh	zh		y	
	[3] s		x=ks	
	[2] z		qu=kwh	
ch	j			
tch	[2] g—			
	—ge			
	dge			

3. Ability to reproduce what is read. This requires ability to choose the most important items in a selection, to summarize and to outline.

4. Ability to locate information through use of an index, a card catalog, atlas and encyclopedia.

TABLE 4.—*The Northampton Charts (Continued)*

Vowel Sounds

¹ OO	² OO	o—e	aw	—o—
(r)u–e		oa	au	
(r)ew		—o (2)	o(r)	
		ow		
ee	—i̇—	a—e	—e— (2)	—a—
—e (1)	–y	ai	ea	
ea		ay		
e–e				
	a(r)	—u—	ur	
		–a	er	
		–ar	ir	
		–er		
		–ir		
		–or		
		–ur		
		–re		

a—e	i—e	o—e	ou (1)	oi	u—e
ai	igh	oa	ow	oy	ew
ay	–y	–o (2)			
		ow			

5. Ability to attack various types of reading material so as to locate facts, to understand sequence or to grasp the general idea.

6. Ability to read with increasing speed.

Even though a teacher has made language preparation for teaching a certain selection in a reader in advance, it is necessary to give guidance in the reading of each selection. In general the lesson may be divided into four parts:

TABLE 5.—*Summary of Word Identification Skills to be Developed through Phonetic and Structural Analysis and Use of Dictionary*

	Primary Grades	Intermediate and Upper Grades
Phonetic Analysis	Teach all spellings of Northampton consonant and vowel charts. Teach blends: Initial: pr tr fr gr dr kr thr br shr sl sp sk sm sn sl sw pl kl fl gl dw kw tw thr str skr spr spl skw Final: st sts ps ks pt kt tn dn nd nt tl dl	Teach all blends: Final: lt lp ls lth lm ldge lch dth dg mpf nth bs gs ls ms vs ths lms thz dths fts sks pts nths bd gd dged thed vd zd ldged tsht tths lfths ndths mpft Teach silent letters: de*b*t Wednesday *s*cene si*gh* *k*new *h*onest ta*l*k island cu*p*board lis*t*en *w*rite
Structural Analysis	Teach spondees: sidewalk, something baseball, etc. Begin instruction in syllabication and accent: 1. Finding first syllable 2. Finding last syllable	Teach suffixes: y ly er est ful less er or ness like eous tion ious able ish ible ant ent age ance ence Prefixes: bi for fore un ex re dis sur in mis ante non com con super pre sub post ab ad trans en inter de pro ex per
Use of Dictionary	Teach order of letters of alphabet. Practice placing familiar words in groups according to first letter of alphabet. Provide practice in finding given word in list beginning with same letter of alphabet.	Teach which one-third or one-fourth of dictionary should be opened to find desired word. Teach alphabetic arrangement according to first three letters of word. Teach use of dictionary as means of: 1. Getting pronunciation of new word: (a) meaning of primary and secondary accents, (b) meaning and use of pronunciation key at bottom of every other page, (c) determining which of two pronunciations of words to choose, (d) how dictionary shows syllabication. 2. Getting meaning of new word: selection of meaning which fits best according to text used. Teach use of special sections: gazetteer, biographic, etc.

1. *Motivation.* The teacher may recall with the children certain experiences of their own which were similar to the one in the book. Pictures may be used to start the discussion. The teacher may tell a portion of the story to arouse interest, but never tells the whole story. The children may look at the illustrations of the selection.

2. *The Assignment.* In the primary grades the teacher and the children read the story together silently either one page, one paragraph or one section at a time. In the intermediate and upper grades the children may be expected to read the entire selection by themselves. This will require that they be supplied with a set of questions to guide their reading. Studies have shown that children retain material better when reading is guided in this way.

3. *The Discussion.* The selection is first discussed in a general way. Children fill out a list of the characters, the setting, the time and the incidents of the story. For little children these generalizations may be listed on the blackboard as, Who:, Where:, When:, and What Happened:. The main incidents are summarized and the climax pointed out. The children may judge the story as humorous, true, imaginary, dull or interesting. The story is then discussed in detail, paragraph by paragraph. Children are asked to locate the more difficult words or strange expressions which the teacher has translated into language familiar to them. The emotional tones, the causal relationships and the why's and how's are noted and talked over.

4. *Checks on Comprehension.* Dramatization is an excellent means of checking comprehension in the primary grades. Dramatization with dialog is especially effective. Deaf children find this a difficult exercise without a script, but can learn with practice to summarize, generalize and use original language through this kind of activity.

Children in the late primary and intermediate and upper grades may be asked to answer a set of questions on the story. Though a few "key" questions as, *Who? Where?* and *How many?* help to orient the children, they are not an effective means of checking on comprehension, because answers to them can be matched mechanically with the text. *Yes* and *no* questions allow for much guessing. *Either/or* questions serve as better checks. Questions which help clarify reasons, feelings and attitudes should be emphasized when checking on comprehension.

The subject of reading cannot be left without referring to the retardation in reading of many deaf children. When reading skills do not develop at a steady pace, the problem of finding suitable reading materials becomes increasingly more difficult as the children grow older and their interests far outdistance their ability to read. Fourteen- and sixteen-year-olds are no longer interested in reading about little white houses for little white rabbits, but are interested in sports, adventure, occupations and probably even in romance. Publishers are becoming more cognizant of the need of furnishing suitable materials for the retarded reader, and appropriate books are appearing in increasing quantities on the market. A series of basic readers has been published in a simplified version, and the juvenile classics have been reduced to levels of difficulty far below the originals.[38, 39] Suggestions for teaching study skills may be found in all the recent textbooks on teaching reading.[33-34, 40-41] Teachers' manuals which accompany the basic readers contain hints which are applicable to teaching deaf children. A good many valuable suggestions on teaching reading to deaf children may be found in current publications.[41-44]

Speech at the Elementary Level

Children who have had preschool training will have the necessary foundation for the more concentrated speech lessons of the elementary school, for they will have gained an understanding of oral communication through having seen speech on the lips and having heard it, though imperfectly through hearing aids. They will have attempted to use their voices in spontaneous vocalization during their play periods, and to communicate orally in halting, partial speech. Some children will even have been mature enough to have been guided into producing a more precise, correct type of speech.

If teachers are aware of the pitfalls which face deaf children in learning to speak they will be better able to give children adequate guidance. Hudgins and Numbers [45] have investigated the intelligibility of the speech of deaf children and have described some general and crucial errors which are made. They found that errors in the production of vowels included neutralization and diphthongization of pure vowels, and substitution of one vowel for another. Failure to close the nasal pharyngeal port imparted a generalized nasal quality to both vowels and consonants in the speech of many deaf children.

Consonant errors were classified under seven categories:

1. The failure to distinguish between voiced and unvoiced sounds. Among the most frequently malarticulated of these sounds were *b, d* and *g.*

2. The substitution of one sound for another: *sh* for *s,* and *w* for *r.*

3. The failure to open the nasal pharyngeal port for the normally resonated sounds *m* and *n,* resulting in substitution of *b* and *d* for them.

4. The malarticulation of blended consonants, as in *six, br*ush and *fl*ower. Here two types of error seem evident: (a) the compound elements fail to fuse because of the slowness of the movements, thereby causing an extraneous vocalization to appear between the two elements, as *sikus* for *six, fulower* for *flower,* (b) one of the elements of the blend is dropped: *skate* becomes *kate* or *sate,* and *chair* becomes *shair.*

5. The malarticulation of abutting consonants. A child may say *note-u-book* for *notebook,* and *in-u-the box* for *in the box.* This sort of error, namely the addition of adventitious syllables, distorts the rhythm of speech.

6. The omission of a consonant at the end of a word, as *daw* for *dog,* and *coa* for *coat.*

7. The omission of a consonant at the beginning of a syllable. The consonants most commonly omitted were *h, l, r, y,* with *th* and *s* being frequent offenders. This last set of errors together with the confusing of voiced and unvoiced sounds and the malarticulation of abutting consonants contributed most to making

the speech of deaf children unintelligible as far as articulatory errors were concerned.

Besides correct articulation and correct accent, phrasing and rhythm were found to be of great importance to intelligibility. Speech which is very slow and labored, as is the speech of many deaf children, loses its characteristic pattern. The sentences spoken with correct rhythm by the children in this study had almost a four to one advantage of being understood over those sentences spoken with incorrect rhythm.

There is definite evidence in Hudgins' further studies to indicate that the speech breathing of deaf children is at a rather primitive level in comparison with that of children who hear, and that deaf children consume considerably more breath while speaking.[46] One of the causes of their excessive use of breath is the maladjustment of the glottis during speech. This results in a breathy tone. The expenditure of an excessive amount of breath on single sounds tends to reduce the length of their phrases and requires the renewal of breath more frequently. Hudgins suggests that an important part of speech training consists in coordinating the movements of the muscles of breathing with the production of the phrase, and that accentuation, grouping and phrasing of syllables should be an inseparable part of speech from the very beginning of instruction.

Besides being able to articulate correctly in rhythmic patterns, deaf children must be able to control the pitch and loudness of their voices. Though poor voice quality may not necessarily affect intelligibility adversely, peculiar inflectional patterns distract, and monotonous, too quiet, harsh or breathy voices are disturbing to listeners.

A glimpse into only a few identifiable "methods" or approaches to teaching speech in the United States might be helpful to the teacher. These methods were devised for elementary aged children in the 1920's or 1930's before nursery school education had become general. They must be appraised in the light of these circumstances.

An approach which attempts to ensure rhythmic speech in children was formulated by Josephine Avondino in the early

1900's.[47, 48] Her method is known as the Babbling Method, a method using syllable drills as the basis for teaching words, phrases or sentences. To ensure smoothness and continuity of speech, work in voice control and proper respiration precedes the practice of syllable drills. To obtain a properly placed voice, the child feels the vibration of tone on the upper and lower part of the teacher's face. The teacher tries to discover the child's best tone, and then works from it while developing the various vowel sounds. The child next imitates prolonged vowels with tones that should approximate those of a hearing child. The consonants are taught separately but no drill is given except in syllables. The basic vowel for the drills is "ah" which is combined with the various consonants to form syllables. They in turn serve as the basis for new words the child is to learn. *Fah* is the basic syllable for monosyllabic words beginning with *f*, *kah* for words beginning with *k*, *tah* for words beginning with *t*, and so on. *Kahfah* are the basic syllables for a two syllable word like *coffee*, containing these consonants. These drills are highly organized so that each child is sure to have practiced all combinations of consonants as releasing and arresting elements in the syllable. They are presented first through imitation. The written form is presented only after the child can imitate the combination from the spoken form automatically.

The system is divided into three stages:

STAGE I. In the formative stage, the consonants are developed in their relation to the vowel sounds in both the initial and final positions. The drills consist of single syllables arranged in groups of threes. They are spoken in succession with natural rapidity.

fah	fah	fah
faw	faw	faw
foo	foo	foo
pah	pah	pah
paw	paw	paw
poo	poo	poo

fah	fah	fah
thah	thah	thah
faw	faw	faw
thaw	thaw	thaw

Before the development of combinations with final *p* and *t,* the development of combinations in the second stage is begun.

STAGE II. Two syllables are combined with the accent falling on the second syllable:

ahfah	ahfah	ahfah
ahfaw	ahfaw	ahfaw
ahpah	ahpah	ahpah
ahpaw	ahpaw	ahpaw

STAGE III. Two syllables each beginning with a consonant are combined with the accent falling on either syllable:

kahfah
kahfaw
kahfoo
kahfee

A new word is introduced through a series of syllable drills. If the word to be taught is *foot,* the child might be required to speak the following series of drills:

fah	fah	fah
faw	faw	faw
fee	fee	fee
foo	foo	foo
faht	faht	faht
fawt	fawt	fawt
feet	feet	feet
foot	foot	foot

This method stresses voice control, breath control and a correct articulation of both vowels and consonants in rhythmic patterns.

The Tadoma Method or Vibration Method was devised by
Kate and Sophia Alcorn [49, 50] who successfully taught several
deaf-blind children (Tad Chapman and Oma Simpson). It was
devised for profoundly deaf children entering school at five years
of age. It is a highly individualized method, since only one or
two children can be taught at a time. This method tries, mainly
by the means of the tactile sense, to present a pattern of speech
which is natural and fluent.

When a child first comes to school, he learns to recognize the
names of objects on the lips. But he also learns to recognize them
through the tactile sense alone. During the first three to five
months the child is saturated with "vibration." He shuts his
eyes while he places his hand lightly on the teacher's cheek in
the area of the mouth. The teacher speaks the name of an object
and the child learns to recognize the spoken form with his eyes
closed, just as a deaf-blind child must. He begins, after some
time, to appreciate the muscular movements associated with
speech, but he is not encouraged, expected, or required to produce voice.

During this same period of three to five months, the breath
consonants are taught through imitation, but all the vowels are
presented in vibration, starting with *oa* as in *boat, ah* as in *father*
and *ou* as in *house*. The child learns the Alcorn Symbols in connection with the work on the vowels. These symbols are abstractions of either the muscular or visual forms of the sounds (see
table 6), and are easily understood as phonetic symbols by even
the youngest children. The children are also taught to recognize
the written form of the vowels using the Northampton Charts
(see table 4).

The child also learns to respond to commands in "vibration,"
such as, *Shut the door, Get your pencil,* and such sentences as *A
boy fell.* A child is encouraged to speak only after he has had
several months of vibration, and especially when the teacher
notices the child's desire to speak. His first utterance may be a
word or a phrase or a single sound. This method claims that
children find a real substitute for the auditory sense by making
use of the tactile and kinesthetic senses, and that not only does

speech become fluent and inflection better, but that lip reading ability and voluntary language is increased.

TABLE 6.—*The Alcorn Symbols (Reproduced with permission of Sophia Alcorn)*

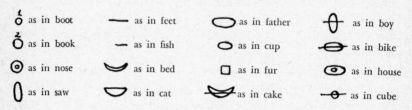

as in boot	as in feet	as in father	as in boy
as in book	as in fish	as in cup	as in bike
as in nose	as in bed	as in fur	as in house
as in saw	as in cat	as in cake	as in cube

The Acoustic Method of Max A. Goldstein,[51] as outlined in the early 1920's, is the precursor of most of the work done in auditory training today. Goldstein advocated the education of the auditory sense long before there were electric hearing aids, and he was one of the first to adopt electric aids in his school—Central Institute for the Deaf in St. Louis. In this method he advocated the interpretation of speech by tactile and auditory impression, to encompass pitch, rhythm, accent, volume and inflection. Though he urged the training of the sense of hearing of all children, his method was used most successfully with children with severe rather than profound losses.

The program consisted of first stimulating the auditory nerve by presenting an organ tone or a pure tone to the child without requiring specific recognition or response. Prolonged vowels on various pitches were then presented. These were spoken directly into the ear, or through a mechanical hearing tube, and after hearing aids were developed they were presented with an amplifier. The teacher held a cardboard between the child's ear and her mouth and was careful not to have bodily contact with the child when she spoke into his ear. The child had to depend on the ear alone for interpretation of what he heard.

Exercises in which a child differentiated between various vowels, as *ah* in *father, o* in *comb, ee* in *key, oo* in *pool* and *ae* in *cake,* followed. He then had to identify and imitate vowels on various pitches as,

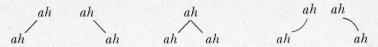

The first consonants presented were *m*— and *n*— in a humming tone. They were combined into syllables with the vowels the child recognized by ear. Other consonants, as *sh, s, f, k, t,* which the child could identify by ear, were combined into syllables to be identified and imitated.

After much of this kind of background drill, phrases and sentences were constructed of the words recognized by ear. The child responded according to the command, direction, question or statement spoken. Accent, phrasing, pitch, inflection and breath control were emphasized in this aspect of the training This pioneer method called attention to the importance of developing the auditory sense in relationship to the speech program.

While the foregoing "methods" all aim to help children develop pleasant, well controlled voices, correct articulation and natural rhythmic speech, they are so structured as to narrow the teacher's approach in solving the problems of the individual child. Much can be learned from them however, and the wise teacher will accept the contributions of these methods in devising her own. In general, the teacher of children with severe and profound hearing losses will do well to teach speech through the multiple sensory approach, using the child's vision, his hearing, his tactile and his kinesthetic senses—all in conjunction with one another. This approach is sometimes referred to as the TVA (tactile, visual, auditory) Method.

Any method which excludes the teaching of rhythmic speech cannot be considered an adequate one. The so-called "Elements Method" in which the phonemes of English are taught as fixed positions, and then strung together without regard to the influence which the various sounds have on each other, is based on a faulty assumption of what speech is. This does not imply, however, that children will not need considerable and expert help in learning to articulate correctly all the elements of speech, or to have guidance in learning to blend one element with another.

In fact, a large part of the teacher's task will be to teach articulation.

The teacher in the elementary school must keep certain principles in mind in the teaching of speech. Perhaps the most important one is this: in order to learn to talk, children must want to talk, must be eager to talk, must love to talk. The only approach to teaching speech must be through encouragement and understanding guidance, not through chastisement or discouragement. Frequently deaf children are unable to grasp speech concepts because they are not clearly presented by the teacher. In her frustration at being unable to get her ideas across, the teacher may shake her head impatiently, look sternly at the child, or even speak crossly to him. No child can be expected to respond favorably to speech under such treatment. Though much repetition, drill and correction are needed for learning the complicated muscular skills involved in speaking, speech lessons must always be pleasurable and rewarding. Another precept to be observed is this: speech development and language growth must proceed as an integrated learning process. Speech drills must be kept meaningful at all times and be related to the language needs of the children. There is a third principle to be kept in mind. Though systematic efforts must be made to guide children into increasing independence and in speaking fluently and correctly, each child must proceed at his own rate. No prescribed order of teaching words, syllables and sounds can be laid down for all children. The speech potential of each child has to be assessed from time to time, and his program on the basis of observed speech behavior.

Objectives for children with severe and profound losses should include the following:

In the Primary Grades: (1) Ability to use clear voice with good glottal adjustment. (2) Ability to adjust the glottis for the aspirate attack. (3) Ability to control loudness and pitch of voice. (4) Ability to use sentence-length breath. (5) Ability to use correct rhythm in sentences and in phrases under the direction of the teacher. (6) Ability to articulate all vowels and consonants correctly in syllables and/or words. (7) Ability to blend sounds correctly (see table 5, page 310). (8) Ability to recognize speech sounds in the written or printed form.

In the Intermediate Grades: (1) Maintenance of good voice quality with conscious control of pitch and loudness. (2) Increasing control over speech breathing processes. (3) Knowledge of rules of accent for polysyllables. (4) Ability to phrase sentences correctly independently. (5) Ability to articulate all initial and final blends.

In the Upper Grades: (1) Maintenance of clear voice with guidance for boys whose voices may change during this period. (2) Mastery of speech breathing process. (3) Ability to speak clearly and intelligibly material of a paragraph or more in length properly phrased and in correct rhythm.

A thorough discussion of techniques of teaching speech to deaf children would require a volume in itself. Therefore, only a few observations on the various aspects of speech training will be made here.

Voice, Pitch, Inflection. The voices of most deaf children are pleasant and natural when they come to school, and every effort should be made to conserve this natural quality. Partially deaf children who use hearing aids effectively usually have no difficulty in maintaining well-placed voices and natural inflection patterns. The profoundly deaf children who do not hear sufficiently to learn voice control through the ear are the ones who require special guidance. The deaf child who can adjust his larynx properly in speaking is likely to have a better voice quality than one who does not. A quick light stroke of the glottis on the initiation of voice is the basis for good voice production. It is equally necessary that a child be able to adjust his glottis for the aspirate attack.[52] He may have to be taught how to make these adjustments consciously before he can differentiate between them and before they become automatic in his speech. Tension in the area of the larynx and pharynx affects voice quality adversely. During the speech lesson the child should always be seated comfortably in a position level with the teacher's face so that no straining or stretching of the head is necessary. Touching a child's larynx may cause a constriction of the laryngeal muscles. A generalized tension may result if too much pressure is put on a child during the lesson, or if the lesson is too long. For more than one reason, short lessons, frequently spaced, are more desirable than one lengthy lesson.

It is entirely possible that a deaf child may enter school with an unnaturally high or low pitched voice. If he cannot be guided into using a desirable pitch through the use of the hearing aid, the approach will have to be through the tactile and kinesthetic senses. The teacher's observation of his spontaneous vocalizations, especially in emotionally charged situations, may give her a clue as to his capacity to vary the pitch of his voice and to produce pleasant tones. If he cannot reproduce these tones in a speech lesson by direct imitation it is possible that he will need a great deal of stimulation through the tactile sense in order to clarify the concept of pitch change. The teacher may frequently hum melodies to him in a clear light voice without expecting an immediate response. When he understands what the teacher is driving at, he may voluntarily hum a tune himself. The teacher may then choose his most pleasant tone and work from that for conscious control of pitch in speech.[53, 54] Some mechanical aids have been constructed which visualize pitch changes for children. In one, lights of different colors flash on when tones of different pitches are produced. Such devices have been found effective with some children when other means have failed.

Loud shrill voices are more easily modified than very soft ones. The child with the quiet voice may be a shy child. All the breath or voice exercises in the world may not convince him that a louder voice is desirable. He must achieve a sense of security in the school situation before the teacher goes to work on his voice problem.

Articulation. Articulation teaching is best begun after a child appreciates the social value of speech. The child who tries to use speech to express his thoughts can better understand the necessity for guidance and correction in speech than one who does not. All articulation teaching should be based on the child's needs and capabilities. If a child can say a whole word or phrase there is no need for his learning its constituent elements before he is allowed to speak such a word. This approach to speech teaching, sometimes referred to as the "Synthetic Method," was described in the section above on the nursery school. It encourages a child to imitate whole words, phrases or sentences. But since there is a limit to the number of words a deaf child can imitate correctly without a knowledge of the individual sounds which make up the words of our language, and since he cannot at first correct his own errors, a time must come when he becomes involved in the difficult task of learning to produce correctly articulated rhythmic speech. Ewing and Ewing [19] recommend that children in nursery school become familiar with the special vocabulary related to the speech apparatus and the act of talking in order to prepare them for articulation teaching in the elementary school. If a child knows such nouns as *mouth, teeth, tongue, lips* and *nose;* such verbs as *blow, flick* and *press;* and such adjectives as *front* and *back,* the relationship of the articulators can be easily explained to him. All the words are first introduced through play experiences before they are directly related to the speech act.

The teacher of the deaf bases her articulation teaching for the individual child on the analysis of the sounds he can produce correctly. These serve as the foundation on which all later speech is built. One new sound is presented at a time. The general principles described in Chapter 7, page 228, for teaching new sounds to the child with moderate losses are entirely applicable to teaching articulation to the deaf. Sufficient provision must be made for the automatic incorporation of the new sound into the child's speech. It must be kept in mind that he has to be guided through certain stages of development until self-correction is made possible through a kinesthetic awareness of the sounds. Only when a child can use a sound automatically in connected speech can it be considered mastered. As soon as he is able to produce a new sound correctly in syllable combinations or with known words, the written form should be associated with it to give him another means of remembering the sound. He should learn all the spellings of the sounds on the Northampton Charts while he is in the primary grades.

Mary New [55] describes a device whereby deaf children may

be helped to distinguish between the voiced, unvoiced and nasal cognates *b p m, d t n* and *g k,* as they occur in the initial position in words. First, the color *red* is associated with the voiced sounds, the color *blue* with the unvoiced and the color *brown* with the nasals. Then all familiar words containing these sounds are classified on charts in which the initial sound is lettered in its appropriate color. Later when the pronunciation is fixed in the child's mind, they are written in the ordinary way. The ingenious teacher is constantly devising such visual aids for teaching speech. Many specific suggestions and techniques for teaching articulation may be found in the references cited in this section.

Rate, Rhythm, Accent and Breath Control. The rate and the rhythm in a deaf child's speech is related to several factors, the language factor being an important one. If a child has to stop to think of the language he is using, his rate will be slowed. He must also be able to control the amount of breath he uses. If he takes a breath after each word, both rate and rhythm will be affected. Deaf children do not need to be taught *how* to breathe, but how to coordinate their breathing with their speech. Sometimes it becomes necessary to teach a child to take in a sufficient amount of breath before he begins to talk, and to practice sentence length-breath with syllable drills, so that he can concentrate on the breath control rather than on the structure of language or on complicated speech patterns. Later this ability has to be transferred to, and practiced with short simple sentences, and then with sentences of increasing length.

Accent is fairly well fixed in those words which a deaf child first learns. The beginnings of accent are usually taught during the rhythm period, and the concept of stress later applied to speech. As soon as a child is ready to learn a word of more than one syllable he must be taught to accent it properly, or again the rhythm of his speech will be distorted. This aspect of speech teaching is closely tied in with articulation teaching. A teacher may want to correct a child who says *ba'bŭ* for *baby* by helping him to pronounce the last syllable as *bee.* She exaggerates the sound in order to call his attention to his error. The child obliges by responding with *babeé*. Unless the child learns immediately to pronounce the word with the correct accent he may forever mispronounce it. Older children frequently have difficulty in imitating the correct accent of polysyllabic words. If this is true the teacher may help to clarify the accent pattern of a word by breaking it up and beginning with the accented syllable. For instance the word *auditorium* would be presented in this way: *to, to*rium, audi*to*rium, or *extravagant* as *trav, trav*agant, ex*trav*agant.

As soon as a child is able to use sentence patterns of more than two words it becomes necessary to teach sentence stress or emphasis. Since emphasis depends largely on meaning, no fixed rules can be taught. The teacher at first guides the child to producing a rhythmic sentence, accenting only the important words —the nouns and verbs. Later the child must learn to group words into phrases and to respect commas and periods as he speaks. Actually, all the aspects of speech—breath control, pitch, inflection, rate, rhythm, articulation and accent—must be taught in a unified approach if deaf children are to have intelligible speech.

Auditory Training and Lip Reading

The one new and rather recent development in the education of children with greatly limited hearing is the use of powerful hearing aids to train the auditory sense. In this area of training lies great hope not only for the child who has considerable residual hearing, but for the one who is profoundly deaf. As has been pointed out in Chapter 6, children with hearing losses do not react to auditory training in a predictable way, but it has been shown that all can benefit from it. Children with extreme losses may or may not show a keen ability to understand speech through the ear alone. Individuals with losses of 85 to 100 db or greater in the speech range have been trained to interpret certain speech patterns sufficiently well to use the telephone in a limited fashion. A child who can dial his home telephone number and recognize his mother's or his father's voice at the other end of the line, and who can deliver a message in intelligible speech, has a skill and an independence which is satisfying and rewarding to him. He may never be able to carry on a conversation with a stranger over a telephone or understand anything but familiar sentence patterns, but the training required to achieve even a little proficiency of this kind is very worth while.

Certain conditions must obtain in order to make the auditory training program effective.

1. Training should begin when the child is very young.

2. The program should be a continuing one throughout his school life.

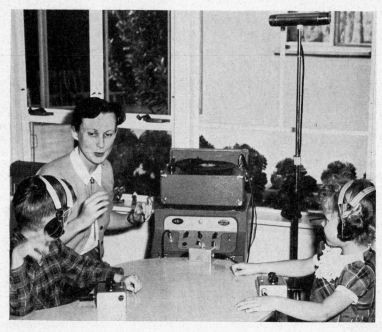

Small remnants of hearing may often be reached with high fidelity, binaural amplification. (Photo courtesy Corvek Medical Equipment Company, Portland, Oregon)

3. It should be carried out as a part of the total educational program. This requires that each classroom be equipped with a group hearing aid and that the aid be used throughout the day, in all instructional activities.

4. The training must be carried out in a suitable environment, that is, in a room in which reverberation is reduced to a minimum and where external and internal room noises are muffled or eliminated.[56]

The person who hears normally learns to ignore background noises but cannot easily interpret speech in a room filled with echoes or in one where the noise level equals or exceeds the level of intensity of speech. And yet this feat is often expected of the untrained deaf ear. Conditions in ordinary classrooms in any but modern schools are usually quite unsatisfactory for auditory training. Since a hearing aid is not capable of selecting the sounds it amplifies, the noises the children hear may be of as great a magnitude as the reverberating speech which they are expected to identify. Every effort must be made to provide a quiet room for auditory training. Room reverberation is reduced by treating ceiling and walls with acoustic materials. Internal noises are controlled by carpeting a room or portions of a room. External noises are largely eliminated by keeping doors and windows tightly shut, by adding double windows to rooms facing noisy thoroughfares and by treating corridors with sound absorbing material. Though the expense of modernizing classrooms is considerable, it seems a folly to invest thousands of dollars in hearing aid equipment without providing an environment in which it can be used effectively.

The teacher's knowledge of how to use hearing aids is also an important element in the auditory training program. She will have to be thoroughly familiar with the operation of the group aid and with its amplifying potentialities. A teacher will find it beneficial to wear a pair of earphones for several days while she is becoming acquainted with it. It goes without saying that she must be responsible for keeping the hearing aid in ready working order. If children are taught to be careful not to drop microphones and earphones and to disconnect them by pulling on the jacks and not on the cords, the care of the aid will be simplified. Extra sets of earphones or cords for individual ear inserts may be kept on hand to replace defective ones. A hearing aid which is not operating properly is not of much value in an auditory training program.

The correct handling of the microphone is vital to good speech reproduction. Most group hearing aids are provided with several hand microphones. All those not in immediate use should be turned off so as to prevent pickup of possible extraneous noises. Microphones in use should not be moved or handled unnecessarily. Speech, to be clearly reproduced, should be delivered close to the microphone. If a speaker wanders away from even a sensitive microphone the volume must be raised so that speech remains audible. If this is not done, possible distortion of speech and an increase of background noise will result. The microphone should be respected as if it were a child's own defective ear. Shouting into it, or moving away from it, does not improve speech reception. It is also important that only one person at a time talk when the hearing aid is in use. Complete confusion results when the hearing aid user is confronted by a babble of voices.

When a teacher and her pupils have agreed on a fairly standardized method of using the group aid, the teacher may proceed to investigate the discriminatory powers of her class; first, in order to help each child arrive at the best possible setting of the controls for his earphones, and then, from time to time, to check on the progress the child is making. These tests may be informal or based on tests devised for the purpose.[57]

A group hearing aid is recommended for the purpose of training of children with severe and profound losses. Auditory training can be conducted with portable table model aids, or even with the child's own wearable aid, if it is done on an individual basis. Unless a teacher respects the rule of staying close to the microphone, she is not really engaged in *training* hearing. Undoubtedly a child who wears his own aid during a class lesson derives some satisfaction from it, for he hears his own voice as he speaks. The other sounds and noises coming to him have the effect of enlivening his environment. This procedure, however, cannot be described as auditory training.

Auditory training should not be considered a school subject, any more than lip reading should be for children with limited hearing. Both are rather the means by which speech and language are perceived. Therefore, the total school program will determine when and to what degree each group of children will learn to discriminate gross sounds, musical sounds and speech.

With a class of primary children whose interests center on *animals,* the auditory training program may be nicely related to this unit of study. For example: A class of six-year-old children was given real experiences with animal pets. One of the children brought his dog to school, and one his cat. The deaf children saw the dog bark and the kitten mew, and heard them over the hearing aid. They held a baby chick, and saw and felt it peep. A few of the children said they heard this sound over the hearing aid. The concept of such vocabulary items as *peep, bark, mew* were developed in this way. They also learned the words, *bow wow, peep peep, meow meow, quack quack, cluck cluck* and the like. They heard recordings of the sounds the animals made. Some of the children were able to recognize these sounds, as well as the words *bow wow, meow meow,* and *peep peep* through the ear alone. Some could identify them only when they looked and listened. Two of the children were never quite sure whether the teacher was speaking unless they were looking at her.

During the rhythm period the children hopped like rabbits and galloped like horses. This they did in accompaniment to piano music.* Recorded songs about animals were provided for the children along with scripts for those who could read. Children listened to these songs and during the speech period learned to "sing" them, not in their entirety, but in parts. In this way auditory training was correlated with the teaching of rhythmic speech. In some schools children are encouraged to listen to recordings during free periods, and in others they listen to them all during the time they are working quietly at their seats while the teacher gives individual instruction to one or two children. This procedure has the effect of alerting children to the fact that sound and not silence is pleasurable. Thus, they learn to enjoy, recognize and "sing" many songs incidentally.

* In some European schools special rooms are equipped for delivering as much as 120 db of sound in a free field. Here children "listen" to music and interpret it according to their impressions. Quite remarkable results have been obtained through such "listening" activities.

In a more advanced grade, a group of ten-year-olds with hearing losses of 90–110 db in the speech range were studying about the beaver. They had visited a conservation exhibit in which beavers were building a dam, and saw movies of beavers at work. The sound track of the movie was used to clarify such words as *crash* and *splash*. The teacher used the hearing aid for all instruction in speech, language and reading, but she also planned exercises especially directed toward increasing the children's ability to listen critically. A paragraph about the beaver was written on the chalkboard. Only familiar vocabulary and language was used. On another section of the chalkboard the teacher had written phrases of different length and accent, as well as pairs of words such as, *swam—tail, branch—saved* and *dam—made,* chosen from the paragraph. The lesson proceeded as follows:

1. The children read the paragraph silently.
2. They watched and listened while the teacher read the entire paragraph from the chalkboard.
3. They looked down while the teacher read the paragraph and raised their hands when she stopped.
4. They looked down while the teacher read a part of the paragraph and told her the last word they had heard her speak.
5. The teacher read the phrases while the children looked and listened.
6. Through hearing alone, the children identified the phrases the teacher read.
7. The teacher read the pairs of words while the children looked and listened.
8. The children, depending on hearing alone, repeated one word of each pair while the teacher pronounced it.

Not all of the children were able to understand everything the teacher said while they depended on listening alone. Whenever a child had difficulty in discriminating what was being said, he had the privilege of looking and listening. The children might not have been able to handle strange material in the same way, nor to recognize the same vocabulary through the ear alone if they had not been thoroughly familiar with the subject.

Through exercises of this kind, however, their limited powers of auditory discrimination were being developed. Suggestions for auditory training may be found in current publications.[58-61]

Lip reading should be as much a part of the integrated program as is auditory training. Occasionally a teacher may wish to plan some parts of a unit of study especially for practice in lip reading, or give a check to see how much the children in her class can understand when they have to depend on their eyes alone. Every time a teacher of the deaf speaks she is really teaching a lesson in lip reading.

CURRICULA IN SCHOOLS FOR THE DEAF

Curriculum practices in schools for the deaf in the United States vary widely. In some schools tradition alone determines the curriculum; in other Regents' examinations, or entrance examinations to Gallaudet College may influence it; in some day schools the curriculum of the regular elementary schools serves as the basis for the school experiences of deaf children. The curriculum in one school may be organized so as to emphasize the three R's; in another, units of work or centers of interest; in a third, core curricula or areas of living; and in many, emphasis is placed on the logical organization of subject matter. Actually the goals in the education of deaf children are essentially those for all children. The modern curriculum attempts to guide children in developing attitudes and gaining knowledge and skills which will help them realize objectives in regard to themselves as individuals, as members of a family and of a social group, as self-sustaining members in the economic community and as citizens devoted to the democratic ideal.

In planning a curriculum for deaf children, one task is to set up goals which present opportunity for orderly and continuing growth of pupils; another, to select those experiences which are best suited to their needs, interests and capabilities; and a third, to make provision for individual differences.

Certain goals will automatically gain precedence in the education of deaf children by virtue of the handicap of deafness itself. If a large part of the school program is devoted to the development of language and speech skills, less time is available for other aspects of the curriculum, unless, of course, the school day or the school year is lengthened. In order that the general goals can be realized to the greatest possible extent, it is necessary to select school experiences very carefully. What these experiences will be is one of the fundamental issues in building the educational program for deaf children. Persistent life situations, those recurring throughout the years from childhood to adulthood which must be dealt with by every member of our society, serve well as a basis for selection.[62] Every person, whether school child or adult, is confronted daily with problems relating to healthful living, food needs, clothing needs, finding satisfactions through friendships and through working in social groups. He comes in contact with plants, animals and insects. He works with tools, machines and household equipment. Every day he deals with physical and chemical forces in his environment. He uses measures and arithmetic computation. He handles money and buys or sells goods. He learns that there is work to be done and that there are laws to be obeyed. Deaf children have much to gain through a program in which persistent life situations are presented over and over again with differing points of view at increasingly mature levels. Each experience becomes the medium through which language and speech is developed. Each serves as the background for further orderly growth, not only of language and vocabulary, but of attitudes, skills and knowledge. These experiences have to be arranged in proper sequence to be of benefit to learners. This approach does not at all exclude the learning of subject matter, but it does imply that subject matter is to be considered a complement to the development of attitudes and skills rather than the means by which knowledge is accumulated.

It has already been pointed out that school experiences of hearing children of a given age may not be entirely suitable for deaf children of the same age, because of the language handicap which extremely limited hearing imposes. For instance, eight- or nine-year-old hearing children are able to engage in complicated discussions about rocket ships and space travel and in arguments about why their fathers are going to vote for a certain presidential candidate. Deaf children of this age will surely have seen comic books or television programs dealing with trips to the moon, and may have worn campaign buttons, but it is doubtful whether their vocabularies and language abilities would allow them even to think about these subjects in verbal terms, much less to discuss them. To illustrate, a nine-year-old deaf boy, looking at the bulletin board on which the pictures of the presidential candidates were displayed, shook his finger at one of them and said: "Bad. Father said he is bad." This child's concept of the use of the word *bad* was definitely limited, and his understanding of politics exceedingly elementary. He is no exception to the rule. Judged by standards for hearing children, deaf children are, in general, retarded educationally from one to four years. These children require a curriculum built to meet their special needs. A watered-down version of the regular curriculum can hardly be considered an adequate one for them.

The factor of retardation presents a real problem in planning a curriculum for deaf children, especially for those in the middle teens who are about to terminate their school experiences, and who are supposed to be ready to take their places in society as wage-earners in a few years. Their interests are the interests of adolescents and young adults, but their verbal abilities may be at the level of ten- or twelve-year-old hearing children. It is of little value to them to know the names of the countries of Africa or even the names of the capitals of the various states, but of great importance to know how to be good workers, good home-makers and good citizens.

Such a group of teen-aged girls had been following a curriculum oriented to a study of subject matter. They were struggling through material which obviously was quite meaningless to them. A program based on "Areas of Living" was planned to take the place of the traditional curriculum during the last three years they were to be in school. It included units on "Home and Family," "Health," "Democratic Group Living" and "Vocations." The girls' interests were challenged from the very beginning. The study started when one of the girls became an aunt, an occasion that created a good deal of interest on the part of the other members of the class. They expressed a desire to learn something about baby-sitting techniques, since several had been called upon to take care of nieces and nephews. The baby-sitting unit grew in scope until it included information about the care and feeding of infants, their illnesses and their growth and development. The girls studied some elementary home nursing in which they learned to make beds properly, how to bathe persons in bed and how to read a thermometer. These activities culminated in a baby party at school for nieces, nephews and neighbor's children. They planned appropriate entertainment and refreshments for the children and their mothers, and everyone had a wonderful time.

In another unit on the home they studied foods, and what constituted well balanced meals. Incidentally they learned to read restaurant menus, and to choose lunches in the school cafeteria that consisted of more than a hot dog, a piece of pie, a piece of cake, an ice cream bar and a soft drink. They also had practice in preparing and serving food properly.

All of the girls made some of their own clothes, having learned to follow a pattern and to use electric sewing machines. One of their projects was to plan how to make their rooms at home more attractive. After a shopping trip to a department store and a visit to a model home, they drew plans for rearranging their furniture, and for organizing their dressers and closets neatly. Some of them actually made changes in their rooms at home as a result of their study. One girl made a dressing table out of orange crates and scrap lumber in order to make her housekeeping easier. She decorated it with a flounce which matched her new curtains, and displayed it proudly to her class when they visited her home.

The unit on "Dating" was a tremendous hit. The girls learned not only how to accept an invitation to a party, but how to refuse one graciously. They read about the fundamentals of good grooming, and decided what clothes were appropriate for various occasions. They organized skits to practice courteous behavior in public places and at social gatherings. They went to a dance as a group at the local Hearing Center and to a restaurant after the dance as the climax to the unit.

On one of their trips they visited the police station, the court house and the city council chambers. They discussed the rules of good citizenship and decided to avoid any unhappy contacts with the law.

All of the girls had had vocational aspirations far beyond their capabilities before they began the unit on "Vocations." They had envisioned themselves as movie stars and airlines hostesses. After much discussion about qualifications for many vocations, after trips to a bakery, a candy factory, a laundry, a dress manufacturing concern, a large office and the vocational school, and after seeing movies dealing with occupations for women, one girl decided she would like to learn photo tinting at the Vocational School. Another wanted to work as a maid in a hospital, and another decided on office work. She actually secured a part time position as a filing clerk on Saturdays. She was able to help the group formulate a list of the personal qualities of a good worker. The girls read want ads, wrote sample letters of application, and had imaginary interviews with employers. They learned how to fill in application blanks for jobs and for Social Security. They calculated salaries based on various hourly wages and had discussions about budgeting these salaries, buying wisely and saving money. The girls participated in the planning of the units and took initiative in making excellent displays for the bulletin boards and in keeping notebooks and records of their activities. These experiences transformed them from indifferent learners to eager participants in group learning and living. Similar programs can be planned for boys or for groups of girls and boys.

Although these girls did not have specific vocational training, they all found jobs as unskilled workers when they left school. Some deaf children, however, show special aptitudes and interests for more skilled types of work. Vocational departments in public residential schools offer specialized training in many kinds of vocations covering agriculture, commercial work, home crafts, semi-professions as barbering, cosmetology, photography, trades and industries, and vocational handicrafts.[2] All the schools do not offer all types of training. Some day schools have affiliations with the local vocational school. Deaf children attend these schools on part time or full time basis working closely with the teacher of the deaf in the language aspects of the program whenever necessary. There is hardly a limit to the kinds of vocations that deaf people have followed. A good vocational training program will have to be based on aptitudes and individual interests, as well as availability of employment.

There are some very bright deaf children whose verbal abilities are outstanding. They are fully capable of following any curriculum, good or bad, and of completing it at the same age as hearing children. Curriculum planners in schools for the deaf are faced with making provisions for these children, as well as for mentally retarded deaf children. It is possible to individualize instruction within the framework of a single curriculum, if it is not a rigid one. Some schools find it more efficacious to provide several curricula, one plan for the brightest, one for the majority and one for the mentally retarded. There is no special desirability in a uniform approach to learning. Each school must determine the needs of its pupils and then, through a constant re-evaluation of the curriculum, provide a rich school life for them.

RECAPITULATION

Children whose severe or profound hearing losses exist from birth or early infancy do not learn language or speech as other children do. They must be taught to communicate by methods especially designed for them. They depend not only on the remnants of their hearing to gain a knowledge of language and speech, but on their visual, tactile and kinesthetic senses. The use of powerful hearing aids has initiated a new era in their education.

The parents' role in training their children is exceedingly important. Parents have it in their power, when their children are very young, to open for them the door to the world of speech and sound. By establishing and maintaining an oral atmosphere in the home, they reinforce what their children are learning in school. The years between two and six are crucial ones for the development of the process of communication in children with limited hearing. An early beginning tends to reduce educational retardation, which results from lack of verbal skill. Because this is so important, provisions have been made in nearly half of all the schools for the deaf in the United States to receive children as pupils at the age of three or three and a half. Most children with severe and profound losses will require the specialized teaching offered in these schools.

A good school program provides experiences for children which ensure their steady growth in knowledge, attitudes and skills, and which satisfy their needs as cooperating members in the family, school and community. In order that children gain clear concepts of the use of language, the teaching of sentence structures, vocabulary, reading and speech must be viewed as an integrated process closely related to the children's experiences. So that children become increasingly independent in the use of language, provision must be made for their active participation in the learning process.

REFERENCES

1. BUREAU OF THE CENSUS, U. S. Department of Commerce, Current Population Report, October 1952.

2. Tabular statement of American schools for the deaf. Am. Ann. Deaf, vol. 99, January 1954.

3. TIMBERLAKE, JOSEPHINE: Lipreader less than a year old. Volta Review 51: 32, January 1949.

4. EWING, IRENE AND EWING, A. W. G.: Opportunity and the Deaf Child. London, University of London Press; Washington, D. C., Volta Bureau, 1947.

5. FIELDER, MIRIAM: Deaf Children in a Hearing World. New York, Ronald Press, 1952.

6. Platform, Recommendations and Pledge to Children (Mid-Century White House Conference on Children and Youth, Inc.). Raleigh, North Carolina, Health Publications Institute, Inc., 1950.

7. POTTER, RALPH; KOPP, GEORGE AND GREEN, HARRIET: Visible Speech. New York, D. Van Nostrand, 1947.

8. AMOSS, HARRY: Ontario School Ability Examination Manual of Directions. Toronto, Ryerson Press, 1936.

9. GUTHRIE, VIRGINIA: A history of preschool education for the deaf. Volta Review 47: 5–9, 56–57, January 1945; 72–76, 116–117, February 1945; 142–146, 186, March 1945.

10. FOREST, ILSE: Early Years at School. New York, McGraw-Hill, 1949.

11. GAY, ROMNEY: Five Little Playmates: A Book of Finger Play. New York, Grosset & Dunlap, 1941.

12. WOODWARD, HELEN: Books for the deaf child. Volta Review 53: 391–399, October 1953.

13. LOWENFELD, BERTHOLD: Creative and Mental Growth. New York, Macmillan, 1947, 1952.

14. LASSMAN, GRACE H.: Language for the Preschool Deaf Child. New York, Grune & Stratton, 1951.

15. MONROE, MARIAN: Growing into Reading. New York, Scott Foresman, 1951.

16. HEIDER, F. AND HEIDER, G.: A comparison of sentence structure of deaf and hearing children. IN Studies in the Psychology of the Deaf. Psychol. Monogr. No. 232, 1940, p. 42 ff.

17. FUSFELD, IRVING: A Cross Section Evaluation of the Academic Programs of Schools for the Deaf. Washington, D. C., Gallaudet College, Bulletin #1, vol. 3, February 1954.

18. PUGH, GLADYS S.: Summaries from "Appraisal of the Silent Reading Abilities of Acoustically Handicapped Children." Am. Ann. Deaf, vol. 91, September 1946.

19. EWING, I. R. AND EWING, A. W. G.: Speech and the Deaf Child. Washington, D. C., Volta Bureau, 1954.

20. NELSON, MYRTHEL: The evolutionary process of methods of teaching language to the deaf with a survey of methods now employed. Am. Ann. Deaf 94: 230–294, May 1944.

21. BARRY, KATHERINE: The Barry System: A System of Objective Language Teaching. Colorado Springs, Gowdy Printing and Engraving Co., 1914.

22. FITZGERALD, EDITH: Straight Language for the Deaf: A System of Instruction for Deaf Children. Austin, Texas, The Stick Company, 1937 (republished by Volta Bureau, 1954).

23. BUELL, EDITH: Outline of Language for Deaf Children (Book I revised and Book II). Washington, D. C., Volta Bureau, 1934, 1954.

24. CROKER, G. W., JONES, M. K. AND PRATT, M. E.: Language Stories and Drills (Books 1–4). 13 Myrtle Street, Brattleboro, Vermont, Vermont Publishing Co., 1939.

25. PUGH, BESSIE: Steps in Language Development for the Deaf: Illustrated in the Fitzgerald Key. Published by the author, 1950.

26. CENTRAL INSTITUTE FOR THE DEAF: Language outline. Am. Ann. Deaf 95: 353–378, September 1950.

27. DAVIES, RACHAEL DAWES: Silent reading but oral English. Volta Review, vol. 50, September 1948.

28. FRIES, C. C.: Teaching and Learning English as a Foreign Language. Ann Arbor, Michigan, University of Michigan Press, 1945.

29. FITZGERALD, MARGARET H.: Vocabulary development for acoustically handicapped children. Am. Ann. Deaf 94: 409–449, November 1949.

30. SHELLGRAIN, EVELYN: Realizing, enriching and anticipating vocabulary for primary deaf classes. Volta Review 56: 62–65, February 1954.

31. NUMBERS, MARY: A word is a word is a word. Volta Review 56: 66–71, February 1954.

32. TIBERIO, CARMEN: Teaching vocabulary in the school shop. Volta Review 56: 75–77, February 1954.

33. BETTS, EMMETT A.: Foundations of Reading Instruction. New York, American Book Co., 1946, p. 70.

34. McKEE, PAUL: The Teaching of Reading. New York, Houghton, Mifflin, 1948.

35. OSTERN, BEATRICE: The use of movie films in a class of the deaf. Volta Review 55: 247, May 1953.

36. HEINL, STELLA ET AL.: A library project to determine the suitability of books for recreational reading of primary grades in the Illinois School for the Deaf. Am. Ann. Deaf 96: 447–542, November 1951.

37. YALE, CAROLINE: Formation and Development of Elementary English Sounds. Northampton, Massachusetts, Clark School for the Deaf, 1946.

38. CROSBY, LAURA: Books of high interest and low vocabulary level to meet the needs of students in grades seven through twelve. Am. Ann. Deaf 93: 339–359, November 1948.

39. Rochester Occupational Reading Series. Syracuse University Press, 920 Irving Ave., Syracuse, New York, 1954.

40. GRAY, WILLIAM: On Their Own in Reading. Chicago, Scott, Foresman, 1948.

41. RUSSELL, DAVID: Children Learn to Read. New York, Ginn & Co., 1949.

42. BENNET, JOSEPHINE: Reading comprehension in the preschool and primary grades. Volta Review 55: 132–136, March 1953.

43. NUMBERS, MARY: Reading in the middle grades. Volta Review 55: 137–140, March 1953.

44. PUGH, GLADYS: Reading for deaf children. Volta Review 50: 426–429, September 1948.

44. ——: Recreational and study type reading. Volta Review 49: 547–582, December 1947.

45. HUDGINS, C. V. AND NUMBERS, F. C.: An investigation of the intelligibility of the speech of the deaf. Genet. Psychol. Monogr. No. 25, 1942, pp. 289–392.

46. HUDGINS, C. V.: The research program in speech at the Clarke School. Volta Review 54: 355–362, October 1952.

47. AVONDINO, JOSEPHINE: The babbling method: A system of syllable drills for natural development of speech. Washington, D. C., Volta Bureau, 1924.

48. ——: Speech as Taught to Beginning Children. IN Proceedings of the Thirty-second Convention of American Instructors of the Deaf. Washington, D. C., U. S. Government Printing Office, 1941.

49. ALCORN, KATE: Speech developed through vibration. Volta Review 40: 633–638, November 1938.

50. ALCORN, SOPHIA: Development of Speech by the Tadoma Method. In Proceedings of the Thirty-second Convention of American Instructors of the Deaf. Washington, D. C., U. S. Government Printing Office, 1941.

51. GOLDSTEIN, MAX A.: The Acoustic Method. St. Louis, The Laryngoscope Press, 1939.

52. HUDGINS, C. V.: Voice production and breath control in the speech of the deaf. Am. Ann. Deaf 82: 338–363, December 1937.

53. HAYCOCK, G. SIBLEY: The Teaching of Speech. Stoke on Trent, England, Hill & Ainsworth, 1933; Washington, D. C., Volta Bureau.

54. CONNERY, JULIA: Voice Building. St. Louis, Central Institute for the Deaf, 1935 (mimeographed).

55. NEW, MARY: Color in speech teaching. Volta Review 44: 133, 199, March–April 1942.

56. HUDGINS, C. V.: Modern hearing aid equipment in schools for the deaf. Volta Review 55: 185–186, April 1953.

57. QUICK, MARIAN: A test for measuring achievement in speech perception among young deaf children. Volta Review 53: 28–31, January 1953.

58. Harris, G.: An acoustic training program for severely deaf children. Volta Review, vol. 48, October 1946: vol. 49, January 1947.

59. PROBYN, JUNE: The training of residual hearing, Volta Review, vol. 43, January–February 1941.

60. WHITEHURST, MARY: Auditory Training for Children. Washington, D. C., Volta Bureau, 1952.

61. ——: Train Your Hearing: Lessons for Practice. Washington, D. C., Volta Bureau, 1947.

62. STRATEMEYER, FLORENCE, FORKNER, HAMDEN, McKIM, MARGARET ET AL.: Developing a Curriculum for Modern Living. New York, Bureau of Publications, Teachers College, Columbia University, 1947.

BIBLIOGRAPHY

General

Tabular Statement of American schools for the deaf. Am. Ann. Deaf, vol. 90, January 1954.

AMOSS, HARRY: Ontario School Ability Examination Manual of Directions. Toronto, Ryerson Press, 1936.

Bureau of the Census. U. S. Department of Commerce, Current Population Report, October 1952.

EWING, IRENE AND EWING, A. W. G.: Opportunity and the Deaf Child. London, University of London Press, 1947; Washington, D. C., Volta Bureau.

FIEDLER, MIRIAM: Deaf Children in a Hearing World. New York, Ronald Press, 1952.

FOREST, ILSE: Early Years at School. New York, McGraw-Hill, 1949.

FUSFELD, IRVING: A Cross Section Evaluation of the Academic Programs of Schools for the Deaf. Washington, D. C., Gallaudet College, Bulletin #1, vol. 3, February 1954.

GAY, ROMNEY: Five Little Playmates: A Book of Finger Play. New York, Grosset & Dunlap, 1941.

GUTHRIE, VIRGINIA: A history of preschool education for the deaf. Volta Review 47: 5–9, 56–57, January 1945; 72–76, 116–117, February 1945; 142–146, 186, March 1945.

HEIDER, F. AND HEIDER, GRACE: A comparison of sentence structure of deaf and hearing children. IN Studies in the Psychology of the Deaf. Psychol. Monogr. No. 232, 1940.

Illinois Annual School for Mothers of Deaf Children: If You Have a Deaf Child. Urbana, Illinois, University of Illinois Press, 1949.

LASSMAN, GRACE: Language for the Preschool Deaf Child. New York, Grune & Stratton, 1951.

LOWENFELD, BERTHOLD: Creative and Mental Growth. New York, Mamillan, 1947, 1952.

Mid-Century White House Conference on Children and Youth, Inc.: Platform and Recommendations and Pledge to Children. Raleigh, North Carolina, Health Publications Institute, Inc., 1950.

MYKLEBUST, HELMER: Your Deaf Child: A Guide for Parents. Springfield, Illinois, C. C. Thomas, 1950.

NELSON, MYRTHEL: The evolutionary process of methods of teaching language to the deaf with a survey of the methods now employed. Am. Ann. Deaf 94: 230–294, May 1949; 354–396, September 1949.

POTTER, RALPH, KOPP, GEORGE AND GREEN, HARRIET: Visible Speech. New York, D. Van Nostrand, 1947.

STRATEMEYER, FLORENCE, FORKNER, HAMDEN, McKIM, MARGARET ET AL.: Developing a Curriculum for Modern Living. New York, Bureau of Publications, Teachers College, Columbia University, 1947.

TIMBERLAKE, JOSEPHINE: Lipreader less than a year old. Volta Review 51: 151, April 1948.

Hearing Aids and Auditory Training

HARRIS, G.: An acoustic training program for severely deaf children. Volta Review, vol. 48, October and December 1946; vol. 49, January 1947.

HUDGINS, C. V.: Modern hearing aid equipment in schools for the deaf. Volta Review, vol. 55, April 1953.

PROBYN, JUNE: The training of residual hearing. Volta Review, vol. 43, January–February 1941.

WHITEHURST, MARY: Auditory Training for Children. Washington, D. C., Volta Bureau, 1952.

——: Train Your Hearing: Lessons for Practice. Washington, D. C., Volta Bureau, 1947.

Language and Vocabulary Techniques

BARRY, KATHERINE: The Barry System: A System of Objective Language Teaching. Colorado Springs, Gowdy Printing & Engraving Co., 1914.

BUELL, EDITH M.: Outline of Language for Deaf Children (Book I revised, Book II). Washington, D. C., Volta Bureau, 1934, 1954.

Central Institute for the Deaf: Language outline. Am. Ann. Deaf 95: 353–378, September 1950.

CROKER, G. W., JONES, M. K. AND PRATT, M. E.: Language Stories and Drills (Books 1–4). Brattleboro, Vermont, Vermont Publishing Co., 1939.

FITZGERALD, EDITH: Straight Language for the Deaf: A System of Instruction for Deaf Children. Austin, Texas, The Stick Co., 1937; Washington, D. C., Volta Bureau, 1954.

FITZGERALD, MARGARET H.: Vocabulary development for acoustically handicapped children. Am. Ann. Deaf 94: 409–449, November 1949.

NUMBERS, MARY: A word is a word is a word. Volta Review 56: 66–71, February 1954.

PUGH, BESSIE: Steps in Language Development for the Deaf (illustrated in the Fitzgerald Key). Published by the author, 1950 (mimeographed).

SHELLGRAIN, EVELYN M.: Realizing, enriching and anticipating vocabulary for primary deaf classes. Volta Review 56: 62–65, February 1954.

TIBERIO, CARMEN S.: Teaching vocabulary in the school shop. Volta Review 56: 75–77, February 1954.

Reading

BENNETT, JOSEPHINE: Reading comprehension in the preschool and primary classes. Volta Review 55: 132–136, March 1953.

BETTS, EMMETT: Foundations of Reading Instruction. New York, American Book Co., 1946, p. 70.

CROSBY, LAURA: Books of high interest and low vocabulary level to meet the needs of students in grades seven through twelve. Am. Ann. Deaf 93: 339–359, November 1948.

GRAY, WILLIAM: On Their Own in Reading. Chicago, Scott Foresman, 1948.

HEINL, STELLA ET AL.: A library project to determine suitability of books for recreational reading of primary grades in the Illinois School for the Deaf. Am. Ann. Deaf 96: 447–466, September 1951; 524–543, November 1951.

MCKEE, PAUL: The Teaching of Reading. New York, Houghton, Mifflin, 1948.

MONROE, MARIAN: Growing into Reading. Chicago, Scott Foresman, 1951.

NUMBERS, MARY E.: Reading in the middle grades. Volta Review 55: 137–140, March 1953.

OSTERN, BEATRICE: The use of movie films in a class of the deaf. Volta Review 55: 247, May 1953.

PUGH, GLADYS S.: Reading for deaf children. Volta Review 50: 426–429, September 1948.

——: Recreational and study-type reading. Volta Review 49: 547–548, 582, December 1947.

——: Summaries from "Appraisal of the Silent Reading Abilities of Acoustically Handicapped Children." Am. Ann. Deaf 91: 33–49, September 1946.

RUSSELL, DAVID: Children Learn to Read. New York, Ginn & Co., 1949.

Syracuse University Press: Rochester Occupational Series. 920 Irving Ave., Syracuse, New York, 1954.

WOODWARD, HELEN: Books for the deaf child. Volta Review 53: 391–399, October 1953.

Speech

ALCORN, KATE: Speech developed through vibration. Volta Review 40: 633–638, November 1938.

ALCORN, SOPHIA: Development of Speech by the Tadoma Method. IN Proceedings of the Thirty-second Convention of American Instructors of the Deaf. Washington, D. C., U. S. Government Printing Office, 1941.

AVONDINO, JOSEPHINE: The Babbling Method: A System of Syllable Drills for Natural Development of Speech. Washington, D. C., Volta Bureau, 1924.

——: Speech as Taught to Beginning Children. IN Proceedings of the Thirty-second Convention of American Instructors of the Deaf. Washington, D. C., U. S. Government Printing Office, 1941.

CONNERY, JULIA: Voice Building. St. Louis, Central Institute for the Deaf, 1935 (mimeographed).

EWING, IRENE AND EWING, A. W. G.: Speech and the Deaf Child. Manchester, England, Manchester University Press; Washington, D. C., Volta Bureau, 1954.

GOLDSTEIN, M. A.: The Acoustic Method. St. Louis, Laryngoscope Press, 1939.

HAYCOCK, G. SIBLEY: The Teaching of Speech. Stoke on Trent, England, Hill & Ainsworth, 1933; Washington, D. C., Volta Bureau.

HUDGINS, C. V.: The research program in speech at Clarke School. Volta Review 54: 355–362, October 1952.

—— AND NUMBERS, F. C.: An investigation of the intelligibility of the speech of the deaf. Genet. Psychol. Monogr. 25: 289–392, 1942.

NEW, MARY: Color in speech training. Volta Review 44: 133, 199, March–April 1942.

YALE, CAROLINE: Formation and Development of Elementary English Sounds. Northampton, Massachusetts, Clarke School for the Deaf, 1946.

Index

345

5613